Zero Point Mastery

The Ultimate 2025 Weight Loss Cookbook

Victor C. Sell

Content

- Encouragement and next steps for continued success

Introduction: The Zero Point Philosophy

Welcome to Zero Point Mastery: The Ultimate 2025 Weight Loss Cookbook a guide designed to help you embark on a transformative journey towards a healthier, happier you. This book is built around the innovative concept of zero-point foods, a key component in achieving sustainable weight loss without sacrificing the joy of eating delicious, satisfying meals.

Overview of the Zero-Point Approach to Weight Loss

The zero-point approach to weight loss is rooted in the idea that not all calories are created equal. Instead of merely counting calories, this method focuses on foods that naturally promote fullness, have lower energy density, and are rich in essential nutrients. These zero-point foods include items like fruits, vegetables, lean proteins, and whole grains, which you can enjoy freely without meticulous tracking.

This approach simplifies meal planning and allows for more flexibility in your diet, making it easier to stick to your weight loss goals. By emphasizing nutrient-dense foods that are naturally low in calories, the zero-point approach helps you maintain a balanced diet while still enjoying a wide variety of delicious meals.

Benefits and Philosophy Behind Zero-Point Foods

Zero-point foods are more than just a list of ingredients; they represent a holistic philosophy towards eating and well-being. Here are some of the core benefits and principles behind incorporating zero-point foods into your diet:

1. Promoting Natural Satiety: Zero-point foods are often high in fiber and protein, which help you feel fuller for longer. This natural satiety helps curb cravings and reduces the likelihood of overeating.

2. Nutrient Density: These foods are packed with essential vitamins, minerals, and antioxidants, supporting overall health and well-being. They nourish your body with the nutrients it needs while keeping calorie intake low.

3. Encouraging a Balanced Diet: The zero-point approach encourages a diverse and balanced diet. By focusing on whole, unprocessed foods, you can enjoy a variety of flavors and textures, making your meals both enjoyable and satisfying.

4. Simplicity and Flexibility: Unlike restrictive diets that require constant counting and measuring, the zero-point philosophy offers a more relaxed approach. You can enjoy a wide range of foods without the stress of calculating every bite, allowing you to focus on the quality and enjoyment of your meals.

5. Supporting Sustainable Weight Loss: By incorporating zero-point foods into your daily routine, you can achieve sustainable weight loss. This method is not about quick fixes but rather about fostering a long-term, healthy relationship with food.

As you journey through this cookbook, you'll discover a wealth of zero-point recipes designed to delight your taste buds and nourish your body. Each chapter will provide practical tips, creative ideas, and delicious meals that align with the zero-point philosophy. Whether you're new to this approach or looking to deepen your understanding, this book is your guide to mastering the art of healthy, delicious, and practical cooking.

Let's embark on this journey together, embracing the power of zero-point foods to transform your life and achieve your weight loss goals. Welcome to Zero Point Mastery a new way of eating, a new way of living.

Getting Started With Zero Points

Embarking on a journey toward healthier eating and weight loss can be both exciting and daunting. The zero-point approach offers a refreshing and manageable way to navigate this journey, focusing on foods that nourish and satisfy without the burden of constant calorie counting. In this chapter, we'll delve into understanding zero-point foods and setting realistic weight loss goals, laying the foundation for a sustainable and enjoyable lifestyle change.

Understanding Zero-Point Foods

Zero-point foods are the cornerstone of this weight loss approach. These foods are considered "zero points" because they are generally low in calories, high in nutrients, and promote satiety. They include a variety of fruits, vegetables, lean proteins, and whole grains. Here's a closer look at what makes these foods so special:

1. Fruits and Vegetables: Most fruits and vegetables are naturally low in calories and rich in vitamins, minerals, and fiber. They are the building blocks of a zero-point diet, offering a wide range of flavors and textures to explore.

2. Lean Proteins: Foods like chicken breast, fish, tofu, and legumes provide essential proteins that help build and repair tissues, support immune function, and keep you feeling full. They are crucial for maintaining muscle mass during weight loss.

3. Whole Grains: Whole grains such as quinoa, brown rice, and oats are nutrient-dense and provide lasting energy. They are an excellent source of fiber, which aids digestion and helps regulate blood sugar levels.

4. Non-Fat Dairy and Eggs: Non-fat Greek yogurt, cottage cheese, and eggs are versatile zero-point foods that can be used in a variety of recipes. They offer protein and important nutrients like calcium and vitamin D.

The key to the zero-point approach is to focus on these wholesome foods, which can be eaten freely, helping you maintain a balanced diet without the need for constant tracking or restriction.

Setting Realistic Weight Loss Goals

Setting realistic and achievable weight loss goals is essential for long-term success. Here's how to approach this important step:

1. Assess Your Starting Point: Begin by evaluating your current health and weight status. Consider factors like body mass index (BMI), waist circumference, and overall fitness level. This assessment will help you understand where you are starting and what goals are reasonable.

2. Define Your Goals: Decide what you want to achieve with your weight loss journey. This could include losing a specific number of pounds, fitting into a particular clothing size, or improving your overall health markers, such as blood pressure or cholesterol levels.

3. Set SMART Goals: Use the SMART criteria to set goals that are Specific, Measurable, Achievable, Relevant, and Time-bound. For example, instead of saying, "I want to lose weight," you might set a goal like, "I want to lose 10 pounds in the next three months by eating zero-point foods and exercising three times a week."

4. Plan for Small Milestones: Break down your larger goal into smaller, manageable milestones. Celebrating these achievements along the way will keep you motivated and provide a sense of accomplishment.

5. Be Kind to Yourself: Remember that weight loss is a journey, and it's normal to experience ups and downs. Be patient and compassionate with yourself, and focus on progress rather than perfection.

6. Monitor and Adjust: Regularly review your progress and adjust your goals as needed. If you find certain strategies aren't working, don't be afraid to try new approaches or seek support from friends, family, or a healthcare professional.

As you begin this journey with zero-point foods, you'll find that this approach not only helps you lose weight but also encourages a healthier, more balanced lifestyle. By understanding the benefits of zero-point foods and setting realistic, achievable goals, you're well on your way to mastering a new way of eating and living. Welcome to a healthier, happier you!

Essential Kitchen Tools for Zero Point Cooking

To make the most of the zero-point approach and create delicious, healthy meals, having the right kitchen tools and a well-organized space is crucial. In this chapter, we will explore the must-have kitchen gadgets and utensils that will simplify your cooking process, as well as provide tips for organizing your kitchen to ensure efficient meal prep.

Must-Have Kitchen Gadgets and Utensils

1. High-Quality Chef's Knife: A sharp, versatile chef's knife is essential for chopping, slicing, and dicing fruits, vegetables, and proteins. A good knife makes meal prep faster and more enjoyable.

2. Cutting Boards: Invest in multiple cutting boards, preferably made of wood or plastic. Use separate boards for fruits and vegetables, raw meats, and cooked foods to prevent cross-contamination.

3. Blender or Food Processor: A powerful blender or food processor is invaluable for making smoothies, sauces, dressings, and purees. It can also help chop vegetables and nuts quickly.

4. Non-Stick Cookware: Non-stick pans and pots are great for cooking with minimal oil, making them perfect for zero-point recipes. Look for high-quality non-stick surfaces that are durable and easy to clean.

5. Baking Sheets and Parchment Paper: Baking sheets are versatile tools for roasting vegetables, baking fish, and more. Lining them with parchment paper can make cleanup easier and prevent sticking.

6. Measuring Cups and Spoons: Accurate measuring tools are essential for following recipes and ensuring portion control. Keep a set of both dry and liquid measuring cups on hand.

7. Spiralizer: A spiralizer allows you to create noodle-like strips from vegetables like zucchini, carrots, and sweet potatoes, making it easy to incorporate more veggies into your meals.

8. Mandoline Slicer: A mandoline slicer can quickly and uniformly slice vegetables and fruits, making it ideal for preparing salads, slaws, and garnishes.

9. Steamer Basket: A steamer basket is a simple tool for steaming vegetables, fish, and more. Steaming preserves nutrients and keeps foods low in fat.

10. Salad Spinner: A salad spinner is perfect for washing and drying leafy greens, ensuring your salads are crisp and not watered down.

11. Grater and Zester: A grater or zester is handy for adding fresh zest from citrus fruits, grating cheese, or finely grating vegetables like carrots or zucchini.

12. Mixing Bowls: A set of mixing bowls in various sizes is useful for preparing ingredients, mixing batters, and serving.

13. Silicone Spatulas: Silicone spatulas are heat-resistant and great for scraping down the sides of bowls and pots, ensuring you make the most of your ingredients.

14. Digital Kitchen Scale: A digital kitchen scale helps with portion control and precise measurements, particularly useful for baking and tracking food intake.

Tips for Organizing Your Kitchen for Efficient Meal Prep

1. Declutter Your Kitchen: Start by decluttering your kitchen and removing items you rarely use. Keep only the essentials within easy reach, and store less frequently used items in cabinets or pantry shelves.

2. Create Zones: Organize your kitchen into zones based on activity, such as a prep area, cooking area, and cleanup area. This organization helps streamline the cooking process and minimizes movement.

3. Keep Essentials Accessible: Store frequently used items, such as knives, cutting boards, and measuring cups, in accessible locations. Use drawer organizers and countertop caddies to keep these tools within reach.

4. Organize Pantry and Refrigerator: Arrange your pantry and refrigerator by category, keeping similar items together. Use clear containers and labels to easily identify contents and avoid food waste.

5. Use Vertical Space: Maximize vertical space by using wall-mounted racks, hooks, and shelves. This is particularly useful for storing pots, pans, utensils, and spices.

6. Prep Ingredients in Advance: Set aside time each week to wash, chop, and store ingredients like vegetables, fruits, and proteins. Having prepped ingredients on hand makes it easier to assemble meals quickly.

7. Invest in Storage Containers: Use airtight containers for storing prepped ingredients, leftovers, and dry goods. Opt for stackable containers to save space and keep your fridge and pantry organized.

8. Keep a Well-Stocked Pantry: Maintain a pantry stocked with zero-point staples like whole grains, legumes, canned vegetables, and spices. This ensures you always have the basics on hand for quick meal preparation.

9. Label and Date: Label and date all stored items, especially in the freezer. This practice helps you keep track of freshness and avoid wasting food.

10. Maintain Cleanliness: Regularly clean your kitchen surfaces, tools, and appliances. A clean kitchen not only promotes food safety but also makes cooking more enjoyable.

By equipping your kitchen with these essential tools and organizing it efficiently, you'll find zero-point cooking to be a seamless and enjoyable part of your daily routine. This preparation will not only save you time and effort but also make it easier to stick to your healthy eating goals.

Zero Point Breakfasts

Starting your day with a nutritious, zero-point breakfast can set the tone for a day of healthy eating and sustained energy. In this chapter, we'll explore energizing morning meals that are not only delicious but also align with the zero-point philosophy. From smoothies to omelets, these recipes will help you kickstart your day on the right note.

1. Berry Banana Smoothie

Ingredients:
- 1 cup fresh or frozen mixed berries (strawberries, blueberries, raspberries)
- 1 banana
- 1 cup unsweetened almond milk
- 1 tablespoon chia seeds
- Ice cubes (optional)

Instructions:
1. Combine all ingredients in a blender.
2. Blend until smooth.
3. Pour into a glass and enjoy immediately.

2. Veggie Egg White Omelet

Ingredients:
- 4 egg whites
- 1/2 cup chopped bell peppers (any color)
- 1/4 cup chopped spinach
- 1/4 cup diced tomatoes
- 1/4 cup sliced mushrooms
- Salt and pepper to taste
- Cooking spray

Instructions:
1. Heat a non-stick skillet over medium heat and spray with cooking spray.
2. Add the bell peppers, spinach, tomatoes, and mushrooms. Sauté until vegetables are tender.

3. Pour egg whites over the vegetables. Season with salt and pepper.

4. Cook until the egg whites are set, then fold the omelet in half and serve.

3. Apple Cinnamon Oatmeal

Ingredients:

- 1/2 cup rolled oats
- 1 cup water or unsweetened almond milk
- 1 apple, diced
- 1/2 teaspoon ground cinnamon
- 1 teaspoon vanilla extract

Instructions:

1. In a pot, bring the water or almond milk to a boil.

2. Add the oats, diced apple, and cinnamon. Reduce heat and simmer for 5-7 minutes, stirring occasionally.

3. Stir in the vanilla extract before serving.

4. Greek Yogurt Parfait

Ingredients:

- 1 cup non-fat Greek yogurt
- 1/2 cup mixed berries
- 1 tablespoon chia seeds
- 1 tablespoon unsweetened shredded coconut (optional)

Instructions:

1. In a bowl or glass, layer the Greek yogurt, berries, chia seeds, and shredded coconut.
2. Repeat the layers until all ingredients are used.
3. Serve immediately.

5. Avocado Toast with Tomato and Basil

<u>*Ingredients*</u>:
- 1 slice whole grain bread
- 1/2 avocado, mashed
- 1/2 tomato, sliced
- Fresh basil leaves
- Salt and pepper to taste

<u>*Instructions*</u>:
1. Toast the whole grain bread until golden brown.
2. Spread the mashed avocado evenly over the toast.
3. Top with tomato slices and fresh basil leaves.
4. Season with salt and pepper before serving.

6. Spinach and Feta Egg Muffins

<u>*Ingredients*</u>:
- 6 egg whites
- 1/2 cup chopped spinach
- 1/4 cup crumbled feta cheese
- 1/4 cup diced red onion
- Salt and pepper to taste
- Cooking spray

**Instructions**:

1. Preheat the oven to 350°F (175°C). Spray a muffin tin with cooking spray.
2. In a bowl, whisk together the egg whites, spinach, feta cheese, and red onion. Season with salt and pepper.
3. Pour the mixture into the muffin tin, filling each cup about two-thirds full.
4. Bake for 15-20 minutes, or until the egg muffins are set.
5. Allow to cool slightly before removing from the tin.

7. Blueberry Banana Pancakes

**Ingredients**:

- 1 banana, mashed
- 1/2 cup rolled oats
- 2 egg whites
- 1/2 teaspoon baking powder
- 1/4 cup fresh blueberries

**Instructions**:

1. In a bowl, mix together the mashed banana, rolled oats, egg whites, and baking powder until well combined.
2. Fold in the blueberries.
3. Heat a non-stick skillet over medium heat. Pour small amounts of the batter into the skillet to form pancakes.
4. Cook for 2-3 minutes on each side, or until golden brown.

8. Chia Pudding

**Ingredients**:

- 1/4 cup chia seeds
- 1 cup unsweetened almond milk
- 1 teaspoon vanilla extract
- Fresh fruit for topping (e.g., berries, mango, kiwi)

Instructions:

1. In a bowl, combine the chia seeds, almond milk, and vanilla extract.
2. Stir well and let sit for about 5 minutes, then stir again to prevent clumping.
3. Cover and refrigerate for at least 2 hours, or overnight.
4. Serve with fresh fruit on top.

9. Sweet Potato and Black Bean Breakfast Bowl

Ingredients:

- 1 small sweet potato, peeled and diced
- 1/2 cup black beans, drained and rinsed
- 1/2 avocado, diced
- 1/4 cup salsa
- Fresh cilantro for garnish
- Salt and pepper to taste

Instructions:

1. Preheat the oven to 400°F (200°C). Place the diced sweet potato on a baking sheet and roast for 20-25 minutes, or until tender.
2. In a bowl, combine the roasted sweet potato, black beans, and avocado.
3. Top with salsa and garnish with fresh cilantro.

4. Season with salt and pepper before serving.

10. Zucchini Noodle Breakfast Bowl

<u>*Ingredients*</u>:
- 1 zucchini, spiralized into noodles
- 1/2 cup cherry tomatoes, halved
- 1/4 cup crumbled feta cheese
- 1 poached egg
- Fresh basil leaves for garnish
- Salt and pepper to taste

<u>*Instructions*</u>:
1. In a non-stick skillet, sauté the zucchini noodles and cherry tomatoes until the noodles are tender.
2. Transfer to a bowl and top with crumbled feta cheese.
3. Add the poached egg on top and garnish with fresh basil leaves.
4. Season with salt and pepper before serving.

These zero-point breakfast recipes are designed to provide you with a healthy and satisfying start to your day. They are easy to prepare and packed with nutrients, making them perfect for anyone looking to enjoy a balanced and delicious breakfast while sticking to their weight loss goals. Enjoy these recipes and explore the endless possibilities of zero-point cooking!

Zero Point Snacks and Appetizers

Having a variety of zero-point snacks and appetizers on hand can help you stay satisfied throughout the day without derailing your healthy eating goals. In this chapter, you'll find quick and healthy recipes for light bites that are perfect for any time of day. These snacks are not only delicious but also packed with nutrients, making them ideal for keeping your energy levels up.

1. Cucumber Hummus Bites

Ingredients:
- 1 large cucumber
- 1/2 cup hummus (any flavor)
- Fresh dill for garnish
- Paprika for sprinkling (optional)

Instructions:
1. Slice the cucumber into thick rounds.
2. Spread a small dollop of hummus on each cucumber slice.
3. Garnish with fresh dill and a sprinkle of paprika, if desired.
4. Serve immediately.

2. Baked Zucchini Chips

Ingredients:
- 2 medium zucchinis, thinly sliced
- Cooking spray

- Salt and pepper to taste
- Optional: garlic powder, paprika, or Italian seasoning for extra flavor

Instructions:

1. Preheat the oven to 225°F (110°C). Line a baking sheet with parchment paper.
2. Arrange the zucchini slices on the baking sheet in a single layer.
3. Lightly spray the zucchini slices with cooking spray and season with salt, pepper, and any optional spices.
4. Bake for 1.5 to 2 hours, flipping halfway through, until the chips are crispy.
5. Allow to cool before serving.

3. Fresh Fruit Salad

Ingredients:

- 1 cup strawberries, hulled and sliced
- 1 cup blueberries
- 1 cup pineapple chunks
- 1 kiwi, peeled and sliced
- Juice of 1 lime
- Fresh mint leaves for garnish

Instructions:

1. In a large bowl, combine the strawberries, blueberries, pineapple, and kiwi.

2. Squeeze the lime juice over the fruit and toss gently to combine.

3. Garnish with fresh mint leaves and serve.

4. Greek Yogurt Dip with Veggies

<u>*Ingredients*</u>:
- 1 cup non-fat Greek yogurt
- 1 tablespoon fresh dill, chopped
- 1 tablespoon fresh parsley, chopped
- 1 clove garlic, minced
- Salt and pepper to taste
- Assorted fresh veggies (carrots, bell peppers, celery, cherry tomatoes) for dipping

<u>*Instructions*</u>:
1. In a small bowl, mix the Greek yogurt with dill, parsley, garlic, salt, and pepper.
2. Serve the dip with an assortment of fresh veggies.

5. Deviled Eggs

<u>*Ingredients*</u>:
- 6 hard-boiled eggs
- 1/4 cup non-fat Greek yogurt
- 1 tablespoon Dijon mustard
- Salt and pepper to taste
- Paprika for garnish

<u>*Instructions*</u>:

1. Cut the hard-boiled eggs in half lengthwise and remove the yolks.
2. In a bowl, mash the yolks with Greek yogurt, Dijon mustard, salt, and pepper until smooth.
3. Spoon or pipe the mixture back into the egg whites.
4. Garnish with paprika and serve.

6. Stuffed Mini Bell Peppers

Ingredients:
- 12 mini bell peppers, halved and seeded
- 1 cup non-fat cottage cheese
- 1/4 cup finely chopped chives
- 1 tablespoon lemon juice
- Salt and pepper to taste

Instructions:
1. In a bowl, mix the cottage cheese with chives, lemon juice, salt, and pepper.
2. Spoon the cottage cheese mixture into the halved mini bell peppers.
3. Arrange on a platter and serve.

7. Apple Nachos

Ingredients:
- 2 apples, thinly sliced
- 2 tablespoons unsweetened almond butter
- 1 tablespoon unsweetened shredded coconut
- 1 tablespoon raisins or chopped dates
- 1 teaspoon ground cinnamon

__Instructions__:
1. Arrange the apple slices on a plate.
2. Drizzle with almond butter and sprinkle with shredded coconut, raisins or chopped dates, and ground cinnamon.
3. Serve immediately.

8. Caprese Skewers

__Ingredients__:
- Cherry tomatoes
- Fresh basil leaves
- Fresh mozzarella balls (mini or bocconcini)
- Balsamic glaze for drizzling

__Instructions__:
1. Skewer a cherry tomato, a basil leaf, and a mozzarella ball onto toothpicks or small skewers.
2. Arrange on a platter and drizzle with balsamic glaze.
3. Serve immediately.

9. Roasted Chickpeas

__Ingredients__:
- 1 can chickpeas, drained and rinsed
- 1 tablespoon olive oil
- 1 teaspoon paprika
- 1/2 teaspoon garlic powder
- Salt and pepper to taste

__Instructions__:

1. Preheat the oven to 400°F (200°C). Line a baking sheet with parchment paper.
2. Toss the chickpeas with olive oil, paprika, garlic powder, salt, and pepper.
3. Spread the chickpeas in a single layer on the baking sheet.
4. Bake for 20-30 minutes, shaking the pan halfway through, until crispy.
5. Allow to cool before serving.

10. Avocado Salsa

Ingredients:
- 2 avocados, diced
- 1/2 red onion, finely chopped
- 1 jalapeño, seeded and finely chopped
- 1 tomato, diced
- Juice of 1 lime
- Salt and pepper to taste
- Fresh cilantro for garnish

Instructions:
1. In a bowl, combine the diced avocados, red onion, jalapeño, and tomato.
2. Squeeze lime juice over the mixture and season with salt and pepper.
3. Garnish with fresh cilantro and serve with vegetable sticks or whole grain crackers.

These zero-point snacks and appetizers are perfect for keeping hunger at bay while staying true to your weight loss goals. Whether you're in need of a quick bite between meals or something light to serve at a gathering, these recipes offer a variety of flavors and textures to enjoy. Happy snacking!

Zero Point Lunches

A satisfying and nutritious lunch can provide the energy you need to power through the rest of your day. This chapter features delicious zero-point lunch recipes, including salad bowls, wraps, and soups, that are both filling and flavorful. These recipes are designed to keep you full and energized without compromising your weight loss goals.

1. Grilled Chicken and Avocado Salad

Ingredients:
- 2 grilled chicken breasts, sliced
- 4 cups mixed greens (spinach, arugula, romaine)
- 1 avocado, diced
- 1 cup cherry tomatoes, halved
- 1/4 cup red onion, thinly sliced
- Juice of 1 lemon
- Salt and pepper to taste

Instructions:
1. In a large bowl, combine the mixed greens, grilled chicken, avocado, cherry tomatoes, and red onion.
2. Drizzle with lemon juice and toss to coat.
3. Season with salt and pepper before serving.

2. Quinoa and Black Bean Bowl

Ingredients:
- 1 cup cooked quinoa
- 1 can black beans, drained and rinsed
- 1 cup corn kernels (fresh or frozen)
- 1 bell pepper, diced
- 1/2 red onion, diced
- 1/2 cup salsa
- Fresh cilantro for garnish

Instructions:
1. In a large bowl, mix the quinoa, black beans, corn, bell pepper, and red onion.
2. Stir in the salsa and mix until well combined.
3. Garnish with fresh cilantro and serve.

3. Tuna and Veggie Lettuce Wraps

Ingredients:
- 1 can tuna packed in water, drained
- 1/2 cup diced cucumber
- 1/4 cup diced bell pepper
- 1/4 cup diced red onion
- 1 tablespoon lemon juice
- Salt and pepper to taste
- Large lettuce leaves (such as romaine or butter lettuce)

Instructions:

1. In a bowl, combine the tuna, cucumber, bell pepper, red onion, and lemon juice.
2. Season with salt and pepper.
3. Spoon the mixture onto lettuce leaves, wrap, and serve.

4. Greek Chickpea Salad

Ingredients:
- 1 can chickpeas, drained and rinsed
- 1 cup cherry tomatoes, halved
- 1 cucumber, diced
- 1/4 cup red onion, thinly sliced
- 1/4 cup Kalamata olives, pitted and halved
- 1/4 cup crumbled feta cheese
- Juice of 1 lemon
- 1 tablespoon olive oil
- Fresh oregano for garnish
- Salt and pepper to taste

Instructions:
1. In a large bowl, combine the chickpeas, cherry tomatoes, cucumber, red onion, olives, and feta cheese.
2. Drizzle with lemon juice and olive oil.
3. Toss to combine and season with salt, pepper, and fresh oregano.
4. Serve immediately or chilled.

5. Turkey and Veggie Roll-Ups

__Ingredients__:
- 4 large slices of turkey breast
- m1/2 cup hummus
- 1 cucumber, julienned
- 1 carrot, julienned
- 1 bell pepper, julienned
- Fresh spinach leaves

__Instructions__:
1. Lay the turkey slices flat and spread a thin layer of hummus on each.
2. Place a few strips of cucumber, carrot, bell pepper, and spinach leaves at one end of each turkey slice.
3. Roll up tightly and secure with toothpicks if needed.
4. Slice each roll-up in half and serve.

6. Lentil and Vegetable Soup

__Ingredients__:
- 1 cup dried lentils, rinsed
- 1 onion, diced
- 2 carrots, diced
- 2 celery stalks, diced
- 1 zucchini, diced
- 4 cups vegetable broth
- 2 cups water
- 1 can diced tomatoes
- 2 cloves garlic, minced
- 1 teaspoon dried thyme
- 1 teaspoon dried oregano

- Salt and pepper to taste

Instructions:
1. In a large pot, sauté the onion, carrots, and celery over medium heat until softened.
2. Add the garlic and cook for another minute.
3. Stir in the lentils, zucchini, vegetable broth, water, diced tomatoes, thyme, and oregano.
4. Bring to a boil, then reduce heat and simmer for 30-35 minutes, or until the lentils are tender.
5. Season with salt and pepper before serving.

7. Mediterranean Stuffed Bell Peppers

Ingredients:
- 4 bell peppers, tops cut off and seeds removed
- 1 cup cooked quinoa
- 1/2 cup chickpeas, drained and rinsed
- 1/2 cup diced tomatoes
- 1/4 cup diced cucumber
- 1/4 cup crumbled feta cheese
- 1 tablespoon olive oil
- Juice of 1 lemon
- Fresh parsley for garnish
- Salt and pepper to taste

Instructions:
1. Preheat the oven to 375°F (190°C).
2. In a bowl, mix the quinoa, chickpeas, tomatoes, cucumber, feta cheese, olive oil, and lemon juice.
3. Season with salt and pepper.

4. Stuff the bell peppers with the quinoa mixture and place them in a baking dish.

5. Cover with foil and bake for 25-30 minutes, or until the peppers are tender.

6. Garnish with fresh parsley before serving.

8. Asian Chicken Salad

Ingredients:

- 2 grilled chicken breasts, sliced
- 4 cups Napa cabbage, shredded
- 1 cup shredded carrots
- 1 bell pepper, thinly sliced
- 1 cup snap peas, halved
- 1/4 cup sliced almonds
- 2 tablespoons sesame seeds
- Fresh cilantro for garnish

Dressing:

- 1/4 cup rice vinegar
- 1 tablespoon soy sauce
- 1 tablespoon honey
- 1 teaspoon sesame oil
- 1 clove garlic, minced
- 1 teaspoon grated ginger

Instructions:

1. In a large bowl, combine the Napa cabbage, carrots, bell pepper, snap peas, sliced almonds, and sesame seeds.

2. Add the grilled chicken slices.

3. In a small bowl, whisk together the dressing ingredients:
rice vinegar, soy sauce, honey, sesame oil, garlic, and ginger.
4. Pour the dressing over the salad and toss to combine.
5. Garnish with fresh cilantro before serving.

9. Spicy Black Bean Soup

<u>Ingredients</u>

- 1 can black beans, drained and rinsed
- 1 onion, diced
- 1 bell pepper, diced
- 2 cloves garlic, minced
- 1 can diced tomatoes with green chilies
- 2 cups vegetable broth
- 1 teaspoon cumin
- 1 teaspoon chili powder
- 1/2 teaspoon smoked paprika
- Salt and pepper to taste
- Fresh cilantro for garnish

<u>Instructions</u>:
1. In a large pot, sauté the onion and bell pepper over medium
heat until softened.
2. Add the garlic and cook for another minute.
3. Stir in the black beans, diced tomatoes with green chilies,
vegetable broth, cumin, chili powder, and smoked paprika.
4. Bring to a boil, then reduce heat and simmer for 15-20
minutes.
5. Season with salt and pepper.
6. Garnish with fresh cilantro before serving.

10. Eggplant and Tomato Stack

Ingredients:
- 1 large eggplant, sliced into rounds
- 2 large tomatoes, sliced
- 1/4 cup fresh basil leaves
- 1/4 cup balsamic vinegar
- 1 tablespoon olive oil
- Salt and pepper to taste

Instructions:
1. Preheat the oven to 400°F (200°C). Line a baking sheet with parchment paper.
2. Arrange the eggplant slices on the baking sheet and brush with olive oil. Season with salt and pepper.
3. Roast for 20-25 minutes, or until the eggplant is tender and golden brown.
4. On a plate, layer the roasted eggplant slices with tomato slices and fresh basil leaves.
5. Drizzle with balsamic vinegar and serve.

These zero-point lunch recipes are designed to be both nutritious and satisfying, offering a range of flavors and textures to keep your midday meals exciting. Whether you're in the mood for a refreshing salad, a hearty soup, or a delicious wrap, these recipes provide plenty of options to suit your tastes and dietary goals. Enjoy these meals and feel good about nourishing your body!

Zero Point Dinners

Dinner is an important meal that can help you unwind and refuel after a long day. This chapter features satisfying zero-point dinners, including hearty main dishes, flavorful sides, and delicious vegetarian options. These recipes are designed to be both filling and healthy, providing a perfect end to your day.

1. Lemon Herb Grilled Chicken

Ingredients:

- 4 boneless, skinless chicken breasts
- Juice of 2 lemons
- 3 cloves garlic, minced
- 1 tablespoon olive oil
- 1 teaspoon dried oregano
- 1 teaspoon dried thyme
- Salt and pepper to taste
- Fresh parsley for garnish

Instructions:

1. In a bowl, combine the lemon juice, garlic, olive oil, oregano, thyme, salt, and pepper.
2. Place the chicken breasts in a resealable bag or shallow dish and pour the marinade over them. Let marinate for at least 30 minutes.

3. Preheat the grill to medium-high heat. Grill the chicken for 6-8 minutes per side, or until fully cooked.
4. Garnish with fresh parsley and serve.

2. Baked Salmon with Asparagus

Ingredients:

- 4 salmon fillets
- 1 bunch asparagus, trimmed
- 2 tablespoons olive oil
- Juice of 1 lemon
- 2 cloves garlic, minced
- Salt and pepper to taste
- Fresh dill for garnish

Instructions:

1. Preheat the oven to 400°F (200°C). Line a baking sheet with parchment paper.
2. Arrange the salmon fillets and asparagus on the baking sheet.
3. Drizzle with olive oil and lemon juice, and sprinkle with garlic, salt, and pepper.
4. Bake for 12-15 minutes, or until the salmon is cooked through and the asparagus is tender.
5. Garnish with fresh dill and serve.

3. Stuffed Bell Peppers

Ingredients:

- 4 bell peppers, tops cut off and seeds removed
- 1 cup cooked quinoa
- 1 can black beans, drained and rinsed
- 1 cup corn kernels
- 1 cup diced tomatoes
- 1 teaspoon cumin
- 1 teaspoon chili powder
- Salt and pepper to taste
- Fresh cilantro for garnish

Instructions:
1. Preheat the oven to 375°F (190°C).
2. In a bowl, mix the quinoa, black beans, corn, diced tomatoes, cumin, chili powder, salt, and pepper.
3. Stuff the bell peppers with the quinoa mixture and place them in a baking dish.
4. Cover with foil and bake for 25-30 minutes, or until the peppers are tender.
5. Garnish with fresh cilantro before serving.

4. Zucchini Noodles with Marinara Sauce

Ingredients:
- 4 medium zucchinis, spiralized into noodles
- 2 cups marinara sauce (store-bought or homemade)
- 1 tablespoon olive oil
- 1 clove garlic, minced
- 1 teaspoon dried basil
- Salt and pepper to taste
- Grated Parmesan cheese for garnish (optional)

Instructions:
1. In a large skillet, heat the olive oil over medium heat. Add the garlic and sauté for 1-2 minutes until fragrant.
2. Add the marinara sauce, dried basil, salt, and pepper. Simmer for 5 minutes.
3. Add the zucchini noodles to the skillet and toss to coat with the sauce. Cook for 2-3 minutes until the noodles are tender.
4. Serve with grated Parmesan cheese, if desired.

5. Cauliflower Fried Rice

Ingredients:
- 1 head cauliflower, grated or riced
- 1 cup mixed vegetables (peas, carrots, corn)
- 2 cloves garlic, minced
- 1 tablespoon soy sauce
- 1 tablespoon sesame oil
- 2 eggs, beaten
- 2 green onions, chopped
- Salt and pepper to taste

Instructions:
1. In a large skillet or wok, heat the sesame oil over medium-high heat. Add the garlic and mixed vegetables, and sauté for 3-4 minutes.
2. Push the vegetables to one side of the skillet and pour the beaten eggs into the empty side. Scramble the eggs until fully cooked, then mix with the vegetables.
3. Add the cauliflower rice and soy sauce, and stir-fry for another 3-4 minutes until the cauliflower is tender.

4. Season with salt and pepper, and garnish with chopped
green onions.

6. Mediterranean Baked Cod

Ingredients:
- 4 cod fillets
- 1 cup cherry tomatoes, halved
- 1/4 cup Kalamata olives, pitted and halved
- 1/4 cup red onion, thinly sliced
- 2 cloves garlic, minced
- 2 tablespoons olive oil
- Juice of 1 lemon
- 1 teaspoon dried oregano
- Salt and pepper to taste
- Fresh parsley for garnish

Instructions:
1. Preheat the oven to 400°F (200°C). Line a baking dish with
parchment paper.
2. Arrange the cod fillets in the baking dish and top with
cherry tomatoes, olives, red onion, and garlic.
3. Drizzle with olive oil and lemon juice, and sprinkle with
oregano, salt, and pepper.
4. Bake for 15-20 minutes, or until the fish is cooked through.
5. Garnish with fresh parsley and serve.

7. Eggplant Parmesan

<u>*Ingredients*</u>:

- 2 large eggplants, sliced into rounds
- 2 cups marinara sauce
- 1 cup shredded mozzarella cheese
- 1/2 cup grated Parmesan cheese
- 1 tablespoon olive oil
- 1 teaspoon dried basil
- Salt and pepper to taste
- Fresh basil for garnish

<u>*Instructions*</u>:

1. Preheat the oven to 375°F (190°C). Line a baking sheet with parchment paper.
2. Arrange the eggplant slices on the baking sheet and brush with olive oil. Season with salt and pepper.
3. Bake for 20-25 minutes, or until the eggplant is tender and golden brown.
4. In a baking dish, layer the eggplant slices with marinara sauce, mozzarella cheese, and Parmesan cheese.
5. Repeat the layers until all ingredients are used, ending with a layer of cheese on top.
6. Bake for 25-30 minutes, or until the cheese is melted and bubbly.
7. Garnish with fresh basil before serving.

8. Chicken and Vegetable Stir-Fry

<u>*Ingredients*</u>:

- 2 chicken breasts, sliced thinly
- 2 cups mixed vegetables (broccoli, bell peppers, snow peas)

- 2 cloves garlic, minced
- 1 tablespoon soy sauce
- 1 tablespoon oyster sauce
- 1 tablespoon olive oil
- 1 teaspoon sesame oil
- Salt and pepper to taste
- Sesame seeds for garnish

Instructions:

1. In a wok or large skillet, heat the olive oil over medium-high heat. Add the garlic and chicken slices, and stir-fry until the chicken is cooked through.
2. Add the mixed vegetables and stir-fry for another 3-4 minutes.
3. Stir in the soy sauce, oyster sauce, and sesame oil. Cook for another 2 minutes, or until the vegetables are tender-crisp.
4. Season with salt and pepper, and garnish with sesame seeds before serving.

9. Vegetarian Stuffed Portobello Mushrooms

Ingredients:

- 4 large portobello mushrooms, stems removed
- 1 cup spinach, chopped
- 1/2 cup cherry tomatoes, diced
- 1/4 cup red onion, finely chopped
- 1/4 cup feta cheese, crumbled
- 1 tablespoon olive oil
- 1 clove garlic, minced
- Salt and pepper to taste

- Fresh parsley for garnish

Instructions:

1. Preheat the oven to 375°F (190°C). Line a baking sheet with parchment paper.

2. In a skillet, heat the olive oil over medium heat. Add the garlic, spinach, cherry tomatoes, and red onion. Sauté until the spinach is wilted and the vegetables are tender.

3. Remove from heat and stir in the feta cheese. Season with salt and pepper.

4. Stuff the mixture into the portobello mushrooms and place them on the baking sheet.

5. Bake for 20-25 minutes, or until the mushrooms are tender.

6. Garnish with fresh parsley and serve.

10. Turkey and Zucchini Meatballs

Ingredients:

- 1 pound ground turkey
- 1 zucchini, grated
- 1/4 cup breadcrumbs (optional)
- 1 egg
- 2 cloves garlic, minced
- 1 teaspoon dried oregano
- 1 teaspoon dried basil
- Salt and pepper to taste
- Marinara sauce for serving

Instructions:

1. Preheat the oven to 400°F (200°C). Line a baking sheet with parchment paper.

2. In a bowl, combine the ground turkey, grated zucchini, breadcrumbs (if using), egg, garlic, oregano, basil, salt, and pepper.
3. Mix until well combined and form into meatballs.
4. Place the meatballs on the baking sheet and bake for 15-20 minutes, or until fully cooked.
5. Serve with marinara sauce and a side of vegetables or salad.

These zero-point dinner recipes are designed to be satisfying and nutritious, offering a variety of flavors and textures to keep your evening meals exciting. Whether you're in the mood for a hearty main dish, a flavorful side, or a delicious vegetarian option, these recipes provide plenty of options to suit

Zero Point Desserts

Indulging in dessert doesn't have to derail your weight loss journey. This chapter features zero-point desserts that are both delicious and guilt-free, allowing you to enjoy a sweet treat without compromising your goals. From fruit-based delights to creamy puddings, these recipes offer satisfying options to satisfy your sweet tooth.

1. Mixed Berry Parfait

Ingredients:

- 1 cup mixed berries (strawberries, blueberries, raspberries)
- 1 cup non-fat Greek yogurt
- 1 teaspoon honey or maple syrup (optional)
- Fresh mint for garnish

Instructions:

1. In a glass or bowl, layer the Greek yogurt with mixed berries.
2. Drizzle with honey or maple syrup, if desired.
3. Garnish with fresh mint and serve.

2. Chia Seed Pudding

Ingredients:

- 1/4 cup chia seeds
- 1 cup unsweetened almond milk
- 1 teaspoon vanilla extract
- 1 tablespoon honey or maple syrup (optional)
- Fresh berries for topping

Instructions:

1. In a bowl, whisk together the chia seeds, almond milk, vanilla extract, and honey or maple syrup.
2. Let sit for 5 minutes, then whisk again to prevent clumping.
3. Cover and refrigerate for at least 2 hours or overnight.
4. Top with fresh berries before serving.

3. Baked Apples with Cinnamon

Ingredients:

- 4 apples, cored
- 1 teaspoon ground cinnamon
- 1 tablespoon honey or maple syrup (optional)
- 1/4 cup water
- Fresh mint for garnish

Instructions:

1. Preheat the oven to 350°F (175°C). Place the apples in a baking dish.
2. Sprinkle the apples with ground cinnamon and drizzle with honey or maple syrup, if desired.
3. Add water to the bottom of the dish and cover with foil.
4. Bake for 20-25 minutes, or until the apples are tender.
5. Garnish with fresh mint and serve warm.

4. Banana Ice Cream

Ingredients:

- 4 ripe bananas, sliced and frozen
- 1 teaspoon vanilla extract
- Optional toppings: fresh berries, dark chocolate chips, nuts

Instructions:

1. In a food processor, blend the frozen banana slices until smooth and creamy.
2. Add the vanilla extract and blend again.

3. Serve immediately with your favorite toppings.

5. *Mango Sorbet*

Ingredients:
- 2 ripe mangoes, peeled and diced
- Juice of 1 lime
- 1 tablespoon honey or maple syrup (optional)

Instructions:
1. Place the mango pieces in a food processor and blend until smooth.
2. Add the lime juice and honey or maple syrup, if desired, and blend again.
3. Transfer the mixture to a container and freeze for at least 2 hours before serving.

6. *Baked Pears with Walnuts*

Ingredients:
- 4 pears, halved and cored
- 1/4 cup walnuts, chopped
- 1 teaspoon ground cinnamon
- 1 tablespoon honey or maple syrup (optional)

Instructions:
1. Preheat the oven to 350°F (175°C). Place the pear halves in a baking dish.

2. Sprinkle the pears with chopped walnuts and ground cinnamon.

3. Drizzle with honey or maple syrup, if desired.

4. Bake for 20-25 minutes, or until the pears are tender.

5. Serve warm.

7. Berry Smoothie Bowl

Ingredients:
- 1 cup mixed berries (frozen)
- 1 banana
- 1/2 cup non-fat Greek yogurt
- 1/2 cup unsweetened almond milk
- Toppings: fresh berries, sliced banana, chia seeds, granola

Instructions:
1. In a blender, combine the mixed berries, banana, Greek yogurt, and almond milk. Blend until smooth.

2. Pour the smoothie into a bowl and top with your favorite toppings.

3. Serve immediately.

8. Chocolate Avocado Pudding

Ingredients:
- 2 ripe avocados
- 1/4 cup unsweetened cocoa powder
- 1/4 cup honey or maple syrup
- 1 teaspoon vanilla extract
- A pinch of salt

- Fresh berries for topping

Instructions:

1. In a food processor, blend the avocados until smooth.
2. Add the cocoa powder, honey or maple syrup, vanilla extract, and salt. Blend until well combined.
3. Chill the pudding in the refrigerator for at least 30 minutes.
4. Serve topped with fresh berries.

9. Grilled Pineapple with Coconut

Ingredients:

- 1 pineapple, peeled, cored, and sliced into rings
- 1/4 cup shredded coconut
- 1 tablespoon honey or maple syrup (optional)
- Fresh mint for garnish

Instructions:

1. Preheat the grill to medium-high heat.
2. Grill the pineapple slices for 2-3 minutes per side, or until grill marks appear.
3. Sprinkle the grilled pineapple with shredded coconut and drizzle with honey or maple syrup, if desired.
4. Garnish with fresh mint and serve warm.

10. Apple and Cinnamon Overnight Oats

<u>*Ingredients*</u>:
- 1/2 cup rolled oats
- 1/2 cup unsweetened almond milk
- 1/2 apple, diced
- 1/2 teaspoon ground cinnamon
- 1 tablespoon honey or maple syrup (optional)
- Fresh apple slices for topping

<u>*Instructions*</u>:
1. In a jar or container, combine the rolled oats, almond milk, diced apple, ground cinnamon, and honey or maple syrup.
2. Stir well and cover. Refrigerate overnight.
3. In the morning, top with fresh apple slices before serving.

These zero-point dessert recipes offer a variety of sweet options that are both delicious and guilt-free. Whether you're in the mood for a creamy pudding, a refreshing sorbet, or a baked fruit treat, these recipes provide satisfying choices to end your meals on a sweet note. Enjoy these desserts while staying on track with your weight loss goals!

The Art of Meal Prepping

Meal prepping is a valuable tool in achieving and maintaining weight loss goals, offering convenience and consistency. This chapter will guide you through planning and preparing meals for the week, as well as efficient grocery shopping and storage tips. Included are 10 meal prep recipes that are easy to make, store well, and are zero-point friendly.

Tips for Meal Prepping

1. Plan Your Meals: Decide on a variety of meals that you can rotate throughout the week to keep things interesting.

2. Make a Shopping List: Write down all the ingredients you need for your chosen recipes and stick to the list to avoid unnecessary purchases.

3. Batch Cooking: Cook large quantities of food that can be portioned out for the week. This saves time and ensures you always have healthy meals ready.

4. Use Proper Storage Containers: Invest in quality containers that are BPA-free, microwave-safe, and leak-proof.

5. Label and Date: Label your containers with the contents and the date they were prepared to keep track of freshness.

10 Zero Point Meal Prep Recipes

1. Turkey and Veggie Lettuce Wraps

<u>**Ingredients**</u>:
- 1 lb ground turkey
- 1 red bell pepper, diced
- 1 zucchini, diced
- 1 carrot, shredded
- 2 cloves garlic, minced
- 1 tablespoon soy sauce
- Lettuce leaves (for wrapping)

- Salt and pepper to taste

Instructions:

1. In a skillet, cook the ground turkey over medium heat until browned.
2. Add the garlic, bell pepper, zucchini, and carrot. Cook until vegetables are tender.
3. Stir in the soy sauce, and season with salt and pepper.
4. Let cool and portion into containers with lettuce leaves for wrapping.

2. Quinoa Salad with Chickpeas and Vegetables

Ingredients:

- 1 cup quinoa, cooked
- 1 can chickpeas, drained and rinsed
- 1 cucumber, diced
- 1 bell pepper, diced
- 1 cup cherry tomatoes, halved
- 1/4 cup red onion, finely chopped
- Juice of 1 lemon
- 2 tablespoons olive oil
- Salt and pepper to taste

Instructions:

1. In a large bowl, combine the cooked quinoa, chickpeas, cucumber, bell pepper, cherry tomatoes, and red onion.
2. Drizzle with lemon juice and olive oil, and season with salt and pepper.

3. Toss well and portion into containers.

3. Chicken and Broccoli Stir-Fry

Ingredients:
- 2 chicken breasts, sliced thinly
- 2 cups broccoli florets
- 1red bell pepper, sliced
- 2 cloves garlic, minced
- 2 tablespoons soy sauce
- 1 tablespoon sesame oil
- Salt and pepper to taste

Instructions:
1. In a wok or skillet, heat the sesame oil over medium-high heat. Add the garlic and chicken slices, and stir-fry until the chicken is cooked through.
2. Add the broccoli and bell pepper, and stir-fry for another 3-4 minutes.
3. Stir in the soy sauce, and season with salt and pepper.
4. Let cool and portion into containers.

4. Egg Muffin Cups

Ingredients:
- 8 eggs
- 1 cup spinach, chopped
- 1/2 cup cherry tomatoes, halved

- 1/2 cup bell pepper, diced
- Salt and pepper to taste

Instructions:

1. Preheat the oven to 350°F (175°C). Grease a muffin tin.
2. In a bowl, whisk the eggs and season with salt and pepper.
3. Divide the spinach, cherry tomatoes, and bell pepper among the muffin cups.
4. Pour the egg mixture over the vegetables.
5. Bake for 15-20 minutes, or until the eggs are set.
6. Let cool and portion into containers.

5. Sweet Potato and Black Bean Bowls

Ingredients:

- 2 large sweet potatoes, diced
- 1 can black beans, drained and rinsed
- 1 red onion, diced
- 1 bell pepper, diced
- 1 teaspoon cumin
- 1 teaspoon chili powder
- Salt and pepper to taste

Instructions:

1. Preheat the oven to 400°F (200°C). Toss the sweet potatoes, red onion, and bell pepper with cumin, chili powder, salt, and pepper.

2. Spread on a baking sheet and roast for 25-30 minutes, or until tender.
3. Mix in the black beans and portion into containers.

6. Balsamic Glazed Salmon and Asparagus

Ingredients:
- 4 salmon fillets
- 1 bunch asparagus, trimmed
- 2 tablespoons balsamic vinegar
- 1 tablespoon olive oil
- 2 cloves garlic, minced
- Salt and pepper to taste

Instructions:
1. Preheat the oven to 400°F (200°C). Place the salmon fillets and asparagus on a baking sheet.
2. In a small bowl, whisk together the balsamic vinegar, olive oil, garlic, salt, and pepper.
3. Drizzle over the salmon and asparagus.
4. Bake for 12-15 minutes, or until the salmon is cooked through and the asparagus is tender.
5. Let cool and portion into containers.

7. Vegetable Soup

Ingredients:

- 2 carrots, sliced
- 2 celery stalks, sliced
- 1 zucchini, diced
- 1 cup green beans, trimmed and cut into pieces
- 1 can diced tomatoes
- 4 cups vegetable broth
- 1 teaspoon dried thyme
- 1 teaspoon dried basil
- Salt and pepper to taste

Instructions:

1. In a large pot, combine all the ingredients.

2. Bring to a boil, then reduce the heat and simmer for 20-25 minutes, or until the vegetables are tender.

3. Let cool and portion into containers.

8. Greek Salad

Ingredients:

- 2 cucumbers, diced
- 2 tomatoes, dice
- 1 red onion, thinly sliced
- 1 bell pepper, diced
- 1/2 cup Kalamata olives, pitted and halved
- 1/2 cup feta cheese, crumbled (optional)
- 2 tablespoons olive oil
- Juice of 1 lemon
- 1 teaspoon dried oregano
- Salt and pepper to taste

Instructions:

1. In a large bowl, combine the cucumbers, tomatoes, red onion, bell pepper, and olives.
2. Drizzle with olive oil and lemon juice, and sprinkle with oregano, salt, and pepper.
3. Toss well and portion into containers.

9. Chicken Fajita Bowls

Ingredients:

- 2 chicken breasts, sliced thinly
- 1 red bell pepper, sliced
- 1 green bell pepper, sliced
- 1 yellow bell pepper, sliced
- 1 red onion, sliced
- 2 tablespoons olive oil
- 1 tablespoon fajita seasoning
- Salt and pepper to taste

Instructions:

1. In a large bowl, toss the chicken, bell peppers, and onion with olive oil and fajita seasoning.
2. Heat a skillet over medium-high heat and cook the chicken and vegetables until the chicken is cooked through and the vegetables are tender.
3. Let cool and portion into containers.

10. Lentil and Veggie Curry

__Ingredients__:

- 1 cup lentils, rinsed
- 2 carrots, diced
- 1 zucchini, diced
- 1 can diced tomatoes
- 1 can coconut milk
- 2 cloves garlic, minced
- 1 tablespoon curry powder
- 1 teaspoon ground turmeric
- Salt and pepper to taste

__Instructions__:

1. In a large pot, combine the lentils, carrots, zucchini, diced tomatoes, coconut milk, garlic, curry powder, turmeric, salt, and pepper.
2. Bring to a boil, then reduce the heat and simmer for 25-30 minutes, or until the lentils are tender.
3. Let cool and portion into containers.

Efficient Grocery Shopping and Storage Tips

1. Plan Ahead: Before heading to the store, create a detailed shopping list based on your meal prep recipes.

2. Buy in Bulk: For items you use frequently, buying in bulk can be cost-effective and reduce packaging waste.

3. Fresh Produce First: Choose fresh fruits and vegetables first, then proceed to the other aisles.

4. Use Reusable Bags: Bring reusable bags to reduce plastic waste and keep your groceries organized.

5. Store Smartly: Label containers with the contents and date, and store them in the refrigerator or freezer according to their shelf life.

6. Prep Ingredients: Wash, chop, and portion out ingredients as soon as you get home to save time during the week.

These meal prep recipes and tips will help you stay on track with your zero-point eating plan, ensuring that you have healthy and delicious meals ready to go. By investing a little time in planning and preparation, you'll make your week easier and more enjoyable!

Zero Point Sauces, Dressings, and Condiments

Adding flavor to your meals doesn't have to mean adding points. This chapter focuses on zero-point sauces, dressings, and condiments that enhance your dishes without compromising your weight loss goals. These homemade recipes are versatile and easy to prepare, offering a delicious way to dress up your meals.

1. Zesty Lemon Herb Dressing

Ingredients:
- Juice of 2 lemons
- 1/4 cup fresh parsley, finely chopped
- 2 tablespoons fresh dill, chopped
- 1 garlic clove, minced
- Salt and pepper to taste

Instructions:
1. In a small bowl, whisk together the lemon juice, parsley, dill, and garlic.
2. Season with salt and pepper to taste.
3. Use as a dressing for salads or a marinade for fish.

2. Creamy Avocado Cilantro Dressing

Ingredients:
- 1 ripe avocado
- 1/4 cup fresh cilantro
- Juice of 1 lime
- 1 garlic clove
- 1/4 cup water
- Salt and pepper to taste

Instructions:
1. In a blender, combine the avocado, cilantro, lime juice, garlic, and water. Blend until smooth.
2. Season with salt and pepper to taste.
3. Use as a dressing for salads or a dip for veggies.

3. Spicy Tomato Salsa

Ingredients:
- 4 ripe tomatoes, diced
- 1/2 red onion, finely chopped
- 1 jalapeño, seeded and minced
- 1/4 cup fresh cilantro, chopped
- Juice of 1 lime
- Salt to taste

Instructions:
1. In a bowl, combine the tomatoes, red onion, jalapeño, cilantro, and lime juice.
2. Season with salt to taste.
3. Serve as a dip with chips or as a topping for tacos and grilled meats.

4. Balsamic Glaze

Ingredients:
- 1 cup balsamic vinegar
- 1 tablespoon honey (optional)

Instructions:
1. In a small saucepan, bring the balsamic vinegar to a simmer over medium heat.
2. Reduce the heat to low and simmer until the vinegar is reduced by half and has thickened, about 15-20 minutes.
3. Stir in honey if desired.

4. Let cool and use as a drizzle over salads, vegetables, or meats.

5. *Garlic Herb Yogurt Dip*

Ingredients:
- 1 cup non-fat Greek yogurt
- 2 cloves garlic, minced
- 2 tablespoons fresh dill, chopped
- 2 tablespoons fresh parsley, chopped
- 1 tablespoon lemon juice
- Salt and pepper to taste

Instructions:
1. In a bowl, mix together the Greek yogurt, garlic, dill, parsley, and lemon juice.
2. Season with salt and pepper to taste.
3. Serve as a dip for vegetables or as a sauce for grilled meats.

6. *Mustard Vinaigrette*

Ingredients:
- 2 tablespoons Dijon mustard
- 1/4 cup apple cider vinegar
- 1 tablespoon honey (optional)
- 1/4 cup water
- Salt and pepper to taste

Instructions:

1. In a small bowl, whisk together the Dijon mustard, apple cider vinegar, honey, and water.
2. Season with salt and pepper to taste.
3. Use as a dressing for salads or as a marinade for chicken.

7. Roasted Red Pepper Sauce

Ingredients:

- 2 red bell peppers, roasted and peeled
- 1 garlic clove
- 1/4 cup fresh basil
- 1 tablespoon olive oil
- Salt and pepper to taste

Instructions:

1. In a blender, combine the roasted red bell peppers, garlic, basil, and olive oil. Blend until smooth.
2. Season with salt and pepper to taste.
3. Use as a sauce for pasta, grilled vegetables, or meats.

8. Cucumber Mint Raita

Ingredients:

- 1 cup non-fat Greek yogurt
- 1/2 cucumber, grated
- 1/4 cup fresh mint, chopped
- 1/2 teaspoon ground cumin
- Salt to taste

__Instructions__:

1. In a bowl, mix together the Greek yogurt, grated cucumber, mint, and ground cumin.

2. Season with salt to taste.

3. Serve as a cooling dip for spicy dishes or as a sauce for grilled meats.

9. Chimichurri Sauce

__Ingredients__:

- 1 cup fresh parsley, finely chopped
- 1/2 cup fresh cilantro, finely chopped
- 2 cloves garlic, minced
- 1/4 cup red wine vinegar
- 2 tablespoons olive oil
- Salt and pepper to taste

__Instructions__:

1. In a bowl, combine the parsley, cilantro, garlic, red wine vinegar, and olive oil.

2. Season with salt and pepper to taste.

3. Use as a marinade or topping for grilled meats and vegetables.

10. Mango Salsa

__Ingredients__:

- 2 ripe mangoes, diced
- 1 red bell pepper, diced
- 1/2 red onion, finely chopped
- 1 jalapeño, seeded and minced
- Juice of 1 lime
- Salt to taste

Instructions:

1. In a bowl, combine the mangoes, red bell pepper, red onion, jalapeño, and lime juice.

2. Season with salt to taste.
3. Serve as a dip with chips or as a topping for fish or chicken.

These zero-point sauces, dressings, and condiments add flavor and variety to your meals without adding unnecessary points. They're perfect for enhancing the taste of salads, grilled meats, vegetables, and more. Enjoy experimenting with these recipes to find your favorite combinations!

Zero Point Drinks and Beverages

Staying hydrated and enjoying flavorful drinks doesn't have to come with added points. This chapter explores a range of zero-point drink options that are refreshing, hydrating, and delicious. From smoothies to teas and infused waters, these beverages are perfect for quenching your thirst while supporting your weight loss goals.

1. Green Detox Smoothie

Ingredients:
- 1 cup spinach
- 1/2 cucumber, peeled and chopped
- 1 green apple, cored and chopped
- Juice of 1 lemon
- 1 cup water

Instructions:
1. In a blender, combine the spinach, cucumber, apple, lemon juice, and water.
2. Blend until smooth.
3. Serve immediately, chilled.

2. Berry Bliss Smoothie

Ingredients:
- 1 cup mixed berries (strawberries, blueberries, raspberries)
- 1/2 banana
- 1 cup unsweetened almond milk
- 1 tablespoon chia seeds

Instructions:
1. Combine the mixed berries, banana, almond milk, and chia seeds in a blender.

2. Blend until smooth.
3. Serve immediately, chilled.

3. Citrus Mint Infused Water

Ingredients:
- 1 orange, sliced
- 1 lemon, sliced
- 1 lime, sliced
- A handful of fresh mint leaves
- 1 liter water

Instructions:
1. In a pitcher, combine the orange, lemon, and lime slices with the mint leaves.
2. Fill the pitcher with water.
3. Refrigerate for at least 2 hours before serving.

4. Ginger Peach Iced Tea

Ingredients:
- 4 black tea bags
- 1-inch piece fresh ginger, sliced
- 2 ripe peaches, sliced
- 4 cups boiling water
- Ice cubes

Instructions:
1. Steep the tea bags and ginger slices in the boiling water for 5-7 minutes.
2. Remove the tea bags and ginger. Add the peach slices.

3. Let the tea cool, then refrigerate until chilled.

4. Serve over ice.

5. Tropical Paradise Smoothie

Ingredients:
- 1 cup pineapple chunks
- 1/2 mango, chopped
- 1/2 banana
- 1 cup coconut water
- A few ice cubes

Instructions:

1. Blend the pineapple, mango, banana, and coconut water until smooth.

2. Add ice cubes and blend again.

3. Serve immediately.

6. Cucumber Lemon Mint Infused Water

Ingredients:
- 1 cucumber, thinly sliced
- 1 lemon, thinly sliced
- A handful of fresh mint leaves
- 1 liter water

Instructions:

1. In a pitcher, combine the cucumber and lemon slices with the mint leaves.

2. Fill the pitcher with water.

3. Refrigerate for at least 2 hours before serving.

7. Berry Hibiscus Iced Tea

Ingredients:
- 4 hibiscus tea bags
- 1 cup mixed berries (strawberries, blueberries, raspberries)
- 4 cups boiling water
- Ice cubes

Instructions:
1. Steep the hibiscus tea bags in the boiling water for 5-7 minutes.
2. Remove the tea bags and add the mixed berries.
3. Let the tea cool, then refrigerate until chilled.
4. Serve over ice.

8. Matcha Green Tea Smoothie

Ingredients:
- 1 teaspoon matcha powder
- 1/2 banana
- 1/2 cup spinach
- 1 cup unsweetened almond milk
- A few ice cubes

Instructions:
1. Blend the matcha powder, banana, spinach, and almond milk until smooth.

2. Add ice cubes and blend again.
3. Serve immediately.

9. Pineapple Mint Infused Water

Ingredients:
- 1 cup pineapple chunks
- A handful of fresh mint leaves
- 1 liter water

Instructions:
1. In a pitcher, combine the pineapple chunks with the mint leaves.
2. Fill the pitcher with water.
3. Refrigerate for at least 2 hours before serving.

10. Apple Cinnamon Detox Water

Ingredients:
- 1 apple, thinly sliced
- 1 cinnamon stick
- 1 liter water

Instructions:
1. In a pitcher, combine the apple slices and cinnamon stick.
2. Fill the pitcher with water.
3. Refrigerate for at least 2 hours before serving.

These zero-point drinks are not only refreshing and hydrating but also packed with natural flavors. Enjoy them as part of your daily routine to stay hydrated and energized while keeping your weight loss journey on track.

Eating Out the Zero Point Way

Dining out can be a challenge when trying to stick to a zero-point eating plan, but it doesn't have to derail your weight loss journey. This chapter offers practical tips for making healthy choices, navigating menus, and managing portion control. Additionally, it includes ten zero-point recipes inspired by popular restaurant dishes, allowing you to enjoy similar flavors at home without the added points.

Tips for Dining Out:

1. Research Ahead: Check the restaurant's menu online and identify zero-point or low-point options.

2. Ask for Modifications: Don't hesitate to ask for dishes to be grilled, steamed, or served without sauces.

3. Portion Control: Consider sharing dishes, ordering appetizers as mains, or taking half your meal home.

4. Beware of Hidden Calories: Watch out for dressings, sauces, and sides that may add unexpected points.

5. Choose Water: Opt for water or unsweetened beverages instead of sugary drinks or alcohol.

Zero Point Recipes Inspired by Dining Out

1. Grilled Chicken Salad

Ingredients:
- 2 boneless, skinless chicken breasts
- Mixed greens (lettuce, spinach, arugula)
- 1 cucumber, sliced
- 1 bell pepper, sliced
- 1/4 cup cherry tomatoes
- 1/4 cup red onion, thinly sliced
- Balsamic vinegar and lemon juice for dressing

Instructions:
1. Grill the chicken breasts until fully cooked, then slice them.
2. Toss the mixed greens with cucumber, bell pepper, cherry tomatoes, and red onion.
3. Top with grilled chicken slices and drizzle with balsamic vinegar and lemon juice.

2. Zucchini Noodles with Marinara

Ingredients:
- 4 zucchini, spiralized
- 2 cups homemade marinara sauce
- Fresh basil leaves for garnish

Instructions:

1. Sauté the zucchini noodles in a non-stick pan until tender.

2. Heat the marinara sauce and pour it over the zucchini noodles.

3. Garnish with fresh basil and serve.

3. Steamed Shrimp and Vegetables

Ingredients:

- 1 lb shrimp, peeled and deveined
- 1 cup broccoli florets
- 1 cup snap peas
- 1 red bell pepper, sliced
- 2 cloves garlic, minced
- Lemon wedges for serving

Instructions:

1. Steam the shrimp and vegetables until the shrimp are pink and the vegetables are tender.

2. Sprinkle with minced garlic and serve with lemon wedges.

4. Cauliflower Fried Rice

Ingredients:

- 1 head cauliflower, grated into rice-sized pieces
- 1 cup mixed vegetables (carrots, peas, bell peppers)
- 2 green onions, sliced
- 2 cloves garlic, minced
- 2 eggs (optional)
- Soy sauce or tamari to taste

<u>*Instructions*</u>:

1. In a large pan, sauté the garlic and mixed vegetables until tender.
2. Add the cauliflower rice and green onions, and cook until heated through.
3. If using eggs, push the mixture to the side and scramble the eggs in the pan.
4. Mix everything together and season with soy sauce or tamari.

5. Greek Yogurt Tzatziki with Veggie Sticks

<u>*Ingredients*</u>:

- 1 cup non-fat Greek yogurt
- 1 cucumber, grated and drained
- 2 cloves garlic, minced
- 1 tablespoon fresh dill, chopped
- Juice of 1 lemon
- Salt and pepper to taste
- Carrot and celery sticks for dipping

<u>*Instructions*</u>:

1. Mix the Greek yogurt, cucumber, garlic, dill, and lemon juice in a bowl.
2. Season with salt and pepper to taste.
3. Serve with carrot and celery sticks.

6. Spicy Grilled Fish Tacos

__Ingredients__:
- 4 white fish fillets (tilapia, cod)
- 1 tablespoon chili powder
- 1 teaspoon cumin
- 1 teaspoon paprika
- 1 teaspoon garlic powder
- Corn tortillas
- Shredded cabbage and salsa for serving

__Instructions__:

1. Mix the chili powder, cumin, paprika, and garlic powder in a small bowl.

2. Rub the spice mix onto the fish fillets and grill until cooked through.

3. Serve the fish in corn tortillas with shredded cabbage and salsa.

7. Mango and Avocado Salsa

__Ingredients__:
- ripe mango, diced
- 1 avocado, diced
- 1/2 red onion, finely chopped
- 1 jalapeño, seeded and minced
- Juice of 1 lime
- Salt and cilantro to taste

__Instructions__:

1. Combine the mango, avocado, red onion, jalapeño, and lime juice in a bowl.

2. Season with salt and cilantro to taste.

3. Serve with grilled chicken or fish.

8. Garlic Herb Mushroom Caps

Ingredients:
- 12 large mushroom caps
- 2 cloves garlic, minced
- 1 tablespoon fresh parsley, chopped
- Olive oil spray
- Salt and pepper to taste

Instructions:
1. Preheat the oven to 375°F (190°C).
2. Place the mushroom caps on a baking sheet and spray with olive oil.
3. Sprinkle with garlic, parsley, salt, and pepper.
4. Bake for 15-20 minutes until tender.

9. Spicy Lentil Soup

Ingredients:
- 1 cup lentils, rinsed
- 1 onion, chopped
- 2 carrots, chopped
- 2 celery stalks, chopped
- 2 cloves garlic, minced
- 1 teaspoon cumin
- 1 teaspoon smoked paprika
- 4 cups vegetable broth

Instructions:

1. In a large pot, sauté the onion, carrots, celery, and garlic
until softened.
2. Add the cumin and smoked paprika and stir.
3. Add the lentils and vegetable broth, bring to a boil, then
simmer until the lentils are tender.
4. Serve hot.

10. Caprese Salad Skewers

***Ingredients*:**
- Cherry tomatoes
- Fresh basil leaves
- Fresh mozzarella balls (bocconcini)
- Balsamic glaze for drizzling

***Instructions*:**
1. Skewer cherry tomatoes, fresh basil leaves, and mozzarella
balls alternately.
2. Drizzle with balsamic glaze before serving.

These recipes allow you to enjoy the flavors and variety of
dining out while staying within your zero-point goals. By
choosing fresh ingredients and simple preparations, you can
create delicious meals that align with your weight loss
journey, even when you're eating out or enjoying
restaurant-inspired dishes at home.

Zero Point Cooking for Families

Adapting zero-point meals for family dinners can be both fun and rewarding. This chapter focuses on creating delicious and healthy meals that the whole family will enjoy, including kid-friendly recipes and tips for involving children in the cooking process. These recipes are designed to appeal to all ages, making it easier to maintain a zero-point lifestyle together.

Tips for Family-Friendly Zero Point Cooking:

1. Involve Kids in Cooking: Let children help with simple tasks like mixing ingredients or assembling dishes.

2. Focus on Familiar Flavors: Use flavors and foods your family already enjoys to introduce new zero-point dishes.

3. Make It Fun: Create themed meals or let kids pick out ingredients at the grocery store.

4. Portion Control and Presentation: Serve meals in fun shapes or on special plates to make them more appealing.

Zero Point Family-Friendly Recipes

1. Turkey and Veggie Stuffed Peppers

Ingredients:

- 4 bell peppers, tops cut off and seeds removed
- 1 lb ground turkey
- 1 onion, chopped
- 1 zucchini, diced
- 1 cup diced tomatoes
- 1 teaspoon garlic powder
- 1 teaspoon Italian seasoning
- Salt and pepper to taste

Instructions:

1. Preheat the oven to 375°F (190°C).
2. In a skillet, cook the ground turkey and onion until browned. Add zucchini and cook until softened.
3. Stir in the diced tomatoes, garlic powder, Italian seasoning, salt, and pepper.
4. Stuff the bell peppers with the turkey mixture and place them in a baking dish.
5. Bake for 20-25 minutes, until the peppers are tender.

2. Zucchini Noodle Spaghetti

Ingredients:

- 4 zucchini, spiralized into noodles
- 1 lb lean ground beef or turkey
- 1 onion, chopped
- 2 cloves garlic, minced
- 1 can (15 oz) crushed tomatoes

- 1 teaspoon Italian seasoning
- Salt and pepper to taste

Instructions:

1. In a skillet, cook the ground meat with onion and garlic until browned.
2. Add the crushed tomatoes and Italian seasoning. Simmer for 10 minutes.
3. Meanwhile, sauté the zucchini noodles in a separate pan until tender.
4. Serve the sauce over the zucchini noodles.

3. Chicken and Veggie Skewers

Ingredients:

- 2 boneless, skinless chicken breasts, cut into cubes
- 1 red bell pepper, cut into chunks
- 1 green bell pepper, cut into chunks
- 1 yellow bell pepper, cut into chunks
- 1 red onion, cut into chunks
- Salt, pepper, and paprika for seasoning

Instructions:

1. Preheat the grill or oven to medium-high heat.
2. Thread the chicken and vegetables onto skewers.
3. Season with salt, pepper, and paprika.
4. Grill or bake for 15-20 minutes, until the chicken is cooked through.

4. Sweet Potato Fries

Ingredients:
- 2 large sweet potatoes, cut into fries
- Olive oil spray
- Salt and pepper to taste
- 1 teaspoon paprika

Instructions:
1. Preheat the oven to 425°F (220°C).
2. Arrange the sweet potato fries on a baking sheet and spray with olive oil.
3. Season with salt, pepper, and paprika.
4. Bake for 25-30 minutes, turning halfway through, until crispy.

5. Mini Veggie Pizzas

Ingredients:
- 4 large portobello mushroom caps, stems removed
- 1 cup tomato sauce
- 1/2 cup cherry tomatoes, halved
- 1/2 cup bell peppers, diced
- 1/4 cup red onion, sliced
- Fresh basil leaves for garnish

Instructions:
1. Preheat the oven to 400°F (200°C).
2. Place the mushroom caps on a baking sheet and spread tomato sauce over each.
3. Top with cherry tomatoes, bell peppers, and red onion.

4. Bake for 10-15 minutes until vegetables are tender.

5. Garnish with fresh basil leaves.

6. Baked Chicken Tenders

Ingredients:
- 1 lb chicken tenders
- 1/2 cup plain non-fat Greek yogurt
- 1 teaspoon garlic powder
- 1 teaspoon paprika
- Salt and pepper to taste

Instructions:

1. Preheat the oven to 400°F (200°C).

2. In a bowl, mix the Greek yogurt, garlic powder, paprika, salt, and pepper.

3. Coat the chicken tenders in the yogurt mixture and place on a baking sheet.

4. Bake for 15-20 minutes, until golden and cooked through.

7. Rainbow Veggie Wraps

Ingredients:
- 4 whole wheat tortillas
- 1 cup hummus
- 1 cup shredded carrots
- 1 cup sliced bell peppers
- 1 cup sliced cucumbers
- 1 cup shredded lettuce
- 1/2 cup cherry tomatoes, halved

<u>*Instructions*</u>:

1. Spread hummus on each tortilla.
2. Layer the vegetables evenly on each tortilla.
3. Roll up tightly and slice in half.

8. *Fruit and Yogurt Parfaits*

<u>*Ingredients*</u>:

- 2 cups non-fat Greek yogurt
- 1 cup mixed berries (strawberries, blueberries, raspberries)
- 1 banana, sliced
- 1 tablespoon honey (optional)

<u>*Instructions*</u>:

1. Layer the Greek yogurt with mixed berries and banana slices in individual serving cups.
2. Drizzle with honey if desired.
3. Serve immediately.

9. *Oven-Baked Veggie Chips*

<u>*Ingredients*</u>:

- 1 zucchini, thinly sliced
- 1 sweet potato, thinly sliced
- 1 beet, thinly sliced
- Olive oil spray
- Salt to taste

Instructions:
1. Preheat the oven to 375°F (190°C).
2. Arrange the sliced vegetables on a baking sheet and spray with olive oil.
3. Sprinkle with salt.
4. Bake for 15-20 minutes, turning halfway through, until crispy.

10. Apple Nachos

Ingredients:
- 2 apples, thinly sliced
- 1 tablespoon peanut butter, melted
- 1 tablespoon Greek yogurt
- 1 tablespoon raisins
- 1 tablespoon chopped nuts (optional)

Instructions:
1. Arrange the apple slices on a plate.
2. Drizzle with melted peanut butter and Greek yogurt.
3. Sprinkle with raisins and chopped nuts if desired.

These zero-point family-friendly recipes make it easy to prepare healthy, delicious meals that everyone will enjoy. By incorporating familiar flavors and fun presentations, you can encourage your family to embrace a zero-point lifestyle, ensuring everyone can benefit from nutritious and satisfying meals.

Navigating Special Diets with Zero Point

Adapting zero-point recipes for various dietary needs can be a rewarding challenge. This chapter focuses on how to tailor your zero-point meals to accommodate vegan, gluten-free, and other dietary restrictions, while still enjoying delicious and nutritious dishes. It includes tips for food substitutions and offers ten versatile recipes suitable for different dietary needs.

Tips for Adapting Zero Point Recipes:

1. Vegan Substitutions: Replace animal products with plant-based alternatives, such as tofu, tempeh, or legumes for protein, and plant-based milk or yogurt.

2. Gluten-Free Options: Use gluten-free grains like quinoa, rice, or gluten-free pasta. Look for gluten-free labels on processed foods.

3. Dairy-Free Alternatives: Use almond milk, coconut milk, or oat milk, and opt for dairy-free yogurt or cheese alternatives.

4. Low-Sodium Choices: Reduce or eliminate added salt and use herbs and spices for flavor.

5. Nut-Free Variations: Substitute nuts with seeds (like sunflower or pumpkin seeds) in recipes calling for nuts.

Zero Point Special Diet Recipes

1. Vegan Lentil and Veggie Stew

Ingredients:
- 1 cup lentils, rinsed
- 1 onion, chopped
- 2 carrots, diced
- 2 celery stalks, diced
- 1 zucchini, diced
- 2 cloves garlic, minced
- 4 cups vegetable broth
- 1 teaspoon cumin
- 1 teaspoon paprika
- Salt and pepper to taste

Instructions:
1. In a large pot, sauté the onion, carrots, celery, and garlic until softened.
2. Add the lentils, zucchini, vegetable broth, cumin, and paprika.

3. Bring to a boil, then reduce heat and simmer for 30-35 minutes until the lentils are tender.
4. Season with salt and pepper.

2. Gluten-Free Quinoa Salad

***Ingredients*:**
- 1 cup quinoa, rinsed
- 2 cups water
- 1 cup cherry tomatoes, halved
- 1 cucumber, diced
- 1 bell pepper, diced
- 1/4 cup red onion, finely chopped
- 1/4 cup fresh parsley, chopped
- Juice of 1 lemon
- Salt and pepper to taste

***Instructions*:**
1. Cook the quinoa in water according to package instructions. Let it cool.
2. In a large bowl, combine the cooled quinoa, cherry tomatoes, cucumber, bell pepper, red onion, and parsley.
3. Drizzle with lemon juice and season with salt and pepper.

3. Dairy-Free Creamy Tomato Soup

***Ingredients*:**
- 4 large tomatoes, chopped
- 1 onion, chopped

- 2 cloves garlic, minced
- 2 cups vegetable broth
- 1/2 cup coconut milk
- 1 teaspoon dried basil
- Salt and pepper to taste

Instructions:

1. In a large pot, sauté the onion and garlic until softened.
2. Add the tomatoes and vegetable broth, and bring to a boil.
3. Reduce heat and simmer for 15-20 minutes.
4. Blend the soup until smooth, then stir in the coconut milk and dried basil.
5. Season with salt and pepper.

4. Vegan Tofu Stir-Fry

Ingredients:

- 1 block firm tofu, cubed
- 1 bell pepper, sliced
- 1 broccoli head, cut into florets
- 1 carrot, julienned
- 2 cloves garlic, minced
- 1 tablespoon soy sauce or tamari
- 1 tablespoon sesame oil (optional for flavor)

Instructions:

1. In a large pan, sauté the tofu cubes until golden brown. Remove and set aside.
2. In the same pan, sauté the bell pepper, broccoli, carrot, and garlic until tender.
3. Add the tofu back to the pan and stir in soy sauce or tamari.

4. Drizzle with sesame oil if desired and serve.

5. Gluten-Free Sweet Potato and Black Bean Tacos

Ingredients:
- 2 large sweet potatoes, diced
- 1 can black beans, drained and rinsed
- 1 teaspoon cumin
- 1 teaspoon chili powder
- Salt and pepper to taste
- Corn tortillas
- Fresh cilantro and lime wedges for garnish

Instructions:
1. Preheat the oven to 400°F (200°C).
2. Toss the sweet potato cubes with cumin, chili powder, salt, and pepper.
3. Spread the sweet potatoes on a baking sheet and roast for 25-30 minutes until tender.
4. In a skillet, heat the black beans and mix in the roasted sweet potatoes.
5. Serve on corn tortillas with fresh cilantro and lime wedges.

6. Nut-Free Hummus

Ingredients:
- 1 can chickpeas, drained and rinsed
- 2 cloves garlic, minced
- Juice of 1 lemon
- 2 tablespoons tahini (substitute sunflower seed butter if avoiding nuts)

- 1 teaspoon cumin
- Salt to taste

Instructions:

1. In a food processor, combine chickpeas, garlic, lemon juice, tahini, and cumin.
2. Blend until smooth, adding water if needed for desired consistency.
3. Season with salt and serve with veggie sticks.

7. Vegan Stuffed Bell Peppers

Ingredients:

- 4 bell peppers, tops cut off and seeds removed
- 1 cup cooked brown rice
- 1 can black beans, drained and rinsed
- 1 cup corn kernels
- 1 onion, chopped
- 1 teaspoon chili powder
- 1 teaspoon cumin
- Salt and pepper to taste

Instructions:

1. Preheat the oven to 375°F (190°C).
2. In a skillet, sauté the onion until softened. Add the rice, black beans, corn, chili powder, and cumin. Season with salt and pepper.
3. Stuff the bell peppers with the rice mixture and place them in a baking dish.
4. Bake for 20-25 minutes until the peppers are tender.

8. Dairy-Free Avocado Chocolate Mousse

Ingredients:
- 2 ripe avocados
- 1/4 cup cocoa powder
- 1/4 cup maple syrup
- 1 teaspoon vanilla extract
- Pinch of salt

Instructions:
1. In a food processor, blend the avocados until smooth.
2. Add the cocoa powder, maple syrup, vanilla extract, and salt.
3. Blend until creamy and well combined.
4. Chill in the refrigerator for at least 30 minutes before serving.

9. Gluten-Free Veggie Frittata

Ingredients:
- 6 eggs
- 1/2 cup almond milk or other dairy-free milk
- 1 cup mixed vegetables (spinach, bell peppers, mushrooms)
- 1 onion, chopped
- Salt and pepper to taste

Instructions:
1. Preheat the oven to 375°F (190°C).

2. In a bowl, whisk the eggs and almond milk. Season with salt and pepper.
3. In an oven-safe skillet, sauté the onion and mixed vegetables until tender.
4. Pour the egg mixture over the vegetables.
5. Bake for 20-25 minutes, until the frittata is set and golden.

10. Vegan Cauliflower Buffalo Wings

Ingredients:
- 1 head cauliflower, cut into florets
- 1 cup chickpea flour
- 1 cup water
- 1 teaspoon garlic powder
- 1 teaspoon paprika
- 1 cup hot sauce (check for vegan and gluten-free)
- 1 tablespoon coconut oil (optional)

Instructions:
1. Preheat the oven to 425°F (220°C).
2. In a bowl, mix chickpea flour, water, garlic powder, and paprika to create a batter.
3. Dip cauliflower florets into the batter and place on a baking sheet.
4. Bake for 20-25 minutes, until crispy.
5. In a small pot, heat the hot sauce and coconut oil, then toss the baked cauliflower in the sauce.

These recipes provide delicious and versatile options for accommodating various dietary needs within a zero-point framework. By making thoughtful substitutions and focusing on fresh, whole ingredients, you can create satisfying meals that cater to vegan, gluten-free, dairy-free, and other special diets while staying aligned with your weight loss goals.

Maintaining Your Weight Loss Journey

Sustaining your weight loss journey requires more than just initial motivation; it involves developing long-term strategies that help you maintain your achievements and continue progressing. This chapter offers practical tips for long-term success, how to navigate plateaus and setbacks, and includes ten recipes that support a sustainable, healthy lifestyle.

Strategies for Long-Term Success:

1. Set Realistic Goals: Focus on achievable milestones and celebrate small victories.

2. Stay Consistent: Stick to your healthy eating and exercise routines, even when progress seems slow.

3. Mindful Eating: Pay attention to hunger and fullness cues, and avoid emotional eating.

4. Adapt and Evolve: Be willing to adjust your strategies as your needs and lifestyle change.

5. Stay Active: Incorporate regular physical activity that you enjoy.

6. Seek Support: Connect with friends, family, or support groups for encouragement and accountability.

7. Handle Setbacks Gracefully: Understand that setbacks are a natural part of the journey and use them as learning opportunities.

Handling Plateaus and Setbacks

Plateaus: When progress slows, try varying your exercise routine, reassessing your diet for hidden calories, or focusing on non-scale victories like improved fitness levels or energy.

Setbacks: If you experience a setback, don't be discouraged. Reflect on what triggered the setback, and plan how to handle similar situations in the future. Return to your healthy habits as soon as possible.

Zero Point Recipes for Sustainability

1. Zero Point Veggie Stir-Fry

<u>*Ingredients*</u>:
- 1 bell pepper, sliced
- 1 carrot, julienned
- 1 zucchini, sliced
- 1 cup broccoli florets
- 1 onion, sliced
- 2 cloves garlic, minced
- 2 tablespoons soy sauce (low sodium)
- 1 tablespoon rice vinegar

<u>*Instructions*</u>:
1. In a large pan, sauté the garlic and onion until fragrant.
2. Add the vegetables and stir-fry until tender-crisp.
3. Stir in soy sauce and rice vinegar.
4. Serve with cauliflower rice or quinoa.

2. Greek Yogurt Chicken Salad

<u>*Ingredients*</u>:
- 2 cups cooked, shredded chicken breast
- 1/2 cup plain non-fat Greek yogurt
- 1 celery stalk, diced
- 1/2 apple, diced
- 1/4 cup red onion, finely chopped

- Salt and pepper to taste

Instructions:
1. In a bowl, mix the Greek yogurt, celery, apple, and red onion.
2. Add the chicken and stir until well combined.
3. Season with salt and pepper.
4. Serve in lettuce wraps or over mixed greens.

3. Lentil and Vegetable Soup

Ingredients:
- 1 cup lentils, rinsed
- 1 onion, chopped 2 carrots, diced
- 2 celery stalks, diced
- 2 cloves garlic, minced
- 1 can diced tomatoes (no salt added)
- 4 cups vegetable broth
- 1 teaspoon thyme
- Salt and pepper to taste

Instructions:
1. In a large pot, sauté the onion, garlic, carrots, and celery until softened.
2. Add the lentils, diced tomatoes, vegetable broth, and thyme.
3. Bring to a boil, then reduce heat and simmer for 30-35 minutes.
4. Season with salt and pepper.

4. Cauliflower Fried Rice

<u>*Ingredients*</u>:

- 1 head cauliflower, grated into rice-sized pieces
- 1 cup mixed vegetables (peas, carrots, corn)
- 2 eggs, beaten
- 2 green onions, chopped
- 2 cloves garlic, minced
- 2 tablespoons soy sauce (low sodium)

<u>*Instructions*</u>:

1. In a pan, scramble the eggs and set aside.
2. Sauté the garlic and green onions, then add the mixed vegetables.
3. Stir in the cauliflower rice and soy sauce.
4. Add the scrambled eggs back into the pan and mix well.

5. Spaghetti Squash with Tomato Basil Sauce

<u>*Ingredients*</u>:

- 1 spaghetti squash
- 2 cups cherry tomatoes, halved
- 1/4 cup fresh basil, chopped
- 2 cloves garlic, minced
- Salt and pepper to taste

<u>*Instructions*</u>:

1. Preheat the oven to 400°F (200°C).
2. Cut the spaghetti squash in half, remove seeds, and bake face down on a baking sheet for 40 minutes.
3. In a pan, sauté the garlic and cherry tomatoes until soft.

4. Scrape the spaghetti squash with a fork to create "noodles" and top with tomato basil sauce.

6. Baked Salmon with Asparagus

Ingredients:
- 4 salmon fillets
- 1 bunch asparagus, trimmed
- 1 lemon, sliced
- 1 teaspoon garlic powder
- Salt and pepper to taste

Instructions:
1. Preheat the oven to 400°F (200°C).
2. Place salmon and asparagus on a baking sheet. Season with garlic powder, salt, and pepper.
3. Top with lemon slices.
4. Bake for 15-20 minutes until the salmon is cooked through.

7. Stuffed Bell Peppers with Quinoa and Black Beans

Ingredients:
- 4 bell peppers, tops cut off and seeds removed
- 1 cup cooked quinoa
- 1 can black beans, drained and rinsed
- 1 cup corn kernels
- 1 teaspoon cumin
- 1 teaspoon chili powder
- Salt and pepper to taste

Instructions:

1. Preheat the oven to 375°F (190°C).
2. Mix the quinoa, black beans, corn, cumin, and chili powder. Season with salt and pepper.
3. Stuff the bell peppers with the mixture and place them in a baking dish.
4. Bake for 25-30 minutes until the peppers are tender.

8. Zoodle Primavera

Ingredients:
- 2 zucchinis, spiralized into noodles
- 1 cup cherry tomatoes, halved
- 1 cup bell peppers, sliced
- 1 cup broccoli florets
- 2 cloves garlic, minced
- 1/4 cup fresh basil, chopped
- Salt and pepper to taste

Instructions:
1. In a pan, sauté the garlic and cherry tomatoes.
2. Add the bell peppers and broccoli, and cook until tender.
3. Stir in the zucchini noodles and fresh basil.
4. Season with salt and pepper and serve.

9. Grilled Chicken with Mango Salsa

Ingredients:
- 4 boneless, skinless chicken breasts
- 1 mango, diced

- 1/2 red onion, diced
- 1/2 red bell pepper, diced
- 1 jalapeño, minced (optional)
- Juice of 1 lime
- Fresh cilantro, chopped
- Salt and pepper to taste

Instructions:

1. Season the chicken breasts with salt and pepper and grill until cooked through.
2. In a bowl, mix the mango, red onion, bell pepper, jalapeño, lime juice, and cilantro.
3. Serve the chicken topped with mango salsa.

10. Berry Chia Pudding

Ingredients:

- 2 cups unsweetened almond milk
- 1/2 cup chia seeds
- 1 cup mixed berries
- 1 teaspoon vanilla extract
- 1 tablespoon maple syrup (optional)

Instructions:

1. In a bowl, mix the almond milk, chia seeds, vanilla extract, and maple syrup.
2. Stir well and refrigerate for at least 2 hours or overnight, until thickened.
3. Serve topped with mixed berries.

These recipes are designed to support a balanced, zero-point lifestyle, helping you maintain your weight loss journey with enjoyable and nutritious meals. Remember, staying consistent and mindful of your choices, adapting to changes, and celebrating your progress will make your journey sustainable and rewarding.

Zero Point Recipes Hacks and Tips

Incorporating zero-point recipes into your daily routine can be both creative and practical. This chapter provides hacks and tips to enhance your recipes, make the most out of leftovers, and minimize waste. It includes ten innovative recipes that showcase these strategies, allowing you to enjoy delicious, healthy meals while being resourceful.

Tips for Enhancing Recipes and Minimizing Waste

1. Batch Cooking: Prepare large quantities of zero-point foods like vegetables and lean proteins, then use them throughout the week.

2. Creative Leftovers: Transform leftovers into new dishes, such as turning roasted veggies into soups or salads.

3. Flavor Boosters: Use herbs, spices, citrus, and vinegars to enhance flavors without adding points.

4. Portion Control: Pre-portion snacks and meals to prevent overeating and reduce waste.

5. Freeze Extras: Freeze leftover meals or ingredients to extend their shelf life.

6. Repurpose Ingredients: Use vegetable scraps for making homemade broths or use overripe fruits in smoothies or baked goods.

7. Smart Storage: Store foods properly to maintain freshness and prevent spoilage.

Zero Point Recipes Hacks

1. Veggie-Packed Frittata Muffins

Ingredients:
- 6 eggs
- 1/2 cup chopped spinach
- 1/2 cup diced bell pepper

- 1/4 cup chopped onion
- 1/4 cup diced tomatoes
- Salt and pepper to taste

Instructions:

1. Preheat oven to 375°F (190°C) and grease a muffin tin.

2. In a bowl, whisk eggs and add vegetables. Season with salt and pepper.

3. Pour the mixture into the muffin tin and bake for 20-25 minutes until set.

4. Use leftover vegetables from previous meals for this recipe.

2. Zucchini Noodle Stir-Fry

Ingredients:

- 2 zucchinis, spiralized into noodles
- 1 cup leftover cooked chicken or tofu
- 1 bell pepper, sliced
- 1/2 onion, sliced
- 2 cloves garlic, minced
- 2 tablespoons soy sauce (low sodium)

Instructions:

1. In a pan, sauté garlic and onion until fragrant.

2. Add bell pepper and cook until tender.

3. Stir in zucchini noodles, leftover chicken or tofu, and soy sauce.

4. Cook for 2-3 minutes until heated through.

3. Stuffed Bell Pepper Quinoa Bowls

Ingredients:
- 2 bell peppers, halved and seeded
- 1 cup cooked quinoa
- 1 can black beans, drained and rinsed
- 1 cup corn kernels
- 1/2 cup salsa
- 1 teaspoon cumin
- Salt and pepper to taste

Instructions:
1. Preheat oven to 375°F (190°C).
2. Mix quinoa, black beans, corn, salsa, and cumin. Season with salt and pepper.
3. Stuff bell pepper halves with the mixture and place in a baking dish.
4. Bake for 20-25 minutes until peppers are tender.
5. Use leftover quinoa and beans from previous meals.

4. Cabbage Wrap Tacos

Ingredients:
- 8 large cabbage leaves
- 1 cup cooked ground turkey or beef (use leftover)
- 1/2 cup diced tomatoes
- 1/4 cup chopped onions
- 1/4 cup shredded lettuce
- Salsa or hot sauce for topping

Instructions:

1. In a pan, reheat the cooked ground turkey or beef.
2. Assemble tacos using cabbage leaves as wraps. Fill with meat, tomatoes, onions, and lettuce.
3. Top with salsa or hot sauce.

5. *Vegetable Broth from Scraps*

Ingredients:

- 2 cups vegetable scraps (onion peels, carrot tops, celery ends, etc.)
- 6 cups water
- 2 cloves garlic
- 2 bay leaves
- Salt and pepper to taste

Instructions:

1. In a large pot, combine vegetable scraps, water, garlic, and bay leaves.
2. Bring to a boil, then simmer for 45-60 minutes.
3. Strain the broth and season with salt and pepper.
4. Use this homemade broth in soups and stews.

6. *Banana Oat Pancakes*

Ingredients:

- 2 ripe bananas
- 1 cup rolled oats
- 2 eggs
- 1 teaspoon vanilla extract
- 1/2 teaspoon cinnamon

Instructions:

1. Blend bananas, oats, eggs, vanilla extract, and cinnamon until smooth.
2. Heat a non-stick skillet and pour batter to form small pancakes.
3. Cook until bubbles form, then flip and cook until golden brown.
4. Use overripe bananas for this recipe.

7. Cauliflower Rice with Leftover Veggies

Ingredients:

- 1 head cauliflower, grated into rice-sized pieces
- 1 cup mixed leftover vegetables
- 1 tablespoon olive oil
- Salt and pepper to taste

Instructions:

1. Heat olive oil in a pan and sauté cauliflower rice for 5 minutes.
2. Add mixed leftover vegetables and stir-fry until heated through.
3. Season with salt and pepper.
4. Great way to use up leftover vegetables.

8. Chickpea Salad Sandwiches

Ingredients:

- 1 can chickpeas, mashed
- 1/4 cup plain non-fat Greek yogurt
- 1 celery stalk, diced

- 1/4 cup red onion, finely chopped
- tablespoon Dijon mustard
- Salt and pepper to taste

Instructions:

1. In a bowl, mix mashed chickpeas, Greek yogurt, celery, red onion, and Dijon mustard.
2. Season with salt and pepper.
3. Serve on whole grain bread or in lettuce wraps.

9. Fruit Salad with Citrus Dressing

Ingredients:

- 2 cups mixed fresh fruit (berries, melon, citrus)
- Juice of 1 orange
- Juice of 1 lime
- 1 tablespoon honey or maple syrup

Instructions:

1. In a bowl, combine mixed fresh fruit.
2. In a small bowl, whisk together orange juice, lime juice, and honey or maple syrup.
3. Pour the dressing over the fruit salad and toss to combine.

10. Roasted Vegetable Soup

Ingredients:

- 4 cups mixed leftover roasted vegetables
- 4 cups vegetable broth
- 1 onion, chopped
- 2 cloves garlic, minced

- 1 teaspoon thyme
- Salt and pepper to taste

Instructions:
1. In a large pot, sauté the onion and garlic until softened.
2. Add the roasted vegetables, vegetable broth, and thyme.
3. Bring to a boil, then simmer for 20 minutes.
4. Blend the soup until smooth and season with salt and pepper.

These recipes and tips help you creatively enhance your zero-point meals while minimizing waste. By using leftovers and maximizing the use of ingredients, you can enjoy a variety of delicious, healthy dishes that support your weight loss journey in a sustainable and resourceful way.

The Science Behind Zero Point Foods

Zero Point Foods are a cornerstone of many weight loss and healthy eating plans because they offer substantial nutritional benefits without adding to your daily points allowance. Understanding the nutritional science behind these foods can help you make informed choices that support your health and weight loss goals.

Nutritional Insights and Health Benefits

1. Rich in Nutrients, Low in Calories: Zero Point Foods are typically nutrient-dense, meaning they provide essential vitamins and minerals while being low in calories. This makes them ideal for weight management.

2. High in Fiber: Many Zero Point Foods, such as fruits, vegetables, and legumes, are high in fiber. Fiber aids digestion, promotes feelings of fullness, and can help regulate blood sugar levels.

3. Protein-Packed: Lean proteins like chicken breast, eggs, and beans are also often Zero Points. Protein is essential for muscle repair, immune function, and overall health, and it helps keep you feeling full longer.

4. Healthy Fats: While fats are generally not Zero Points, many Zero Point Foods contain small amounts of healthy fats, like those in fish, which are rich in omega-3 fatty acids that benefit heart health.

5. Hydrating: Many fruits and vegetables are high in water content, helping to keep you hydrated and support metabolic processes.

6. Antioxidants: Zero Point Foods often contain antioxidants, which help combat oxidative stress in the body and can reduce the risk of chronic diseases.

Understanding Macronutrients and Micronutrients

Macronutrients: These include carbohydrates, proteins, and fats. Zero Point Foods primarily focus on providing complex carbohydrates (like those found in vegetables and legumes), lean proteins, and minimal fats.

Micronutrients: These include vitamins and minerals such as vitamin C, potassium, and iron. Zero Point Foods are often rich in these nutrients, supporting overall health.

Zero Point Recipes Highlighting Nutritional Benefits

1. Spinach and Tomato Omelet

Ingredients:
- 2 eggs

- 1 cup spinach, chopped
- 1/2 cup cherry tomatoes, halved
- Salt and pepper to taste

Instructions:

1. In a bowl, beat the eggs and season with salt and pepper.
2. In a non-stick pan, sauté spinach and tomatoes until wilted.
3. Pour the eggs over the vegetables and cook until set.
4. Fold and serve.

Nutritional Insight: High in protein and packed with vitamins A and C from spinach and tomatoes.

2. Chickpea and Cucumber Salad

Ingredients:

- 1 can chickpeas, drained and rinsed
- 1 cucumber, diced
- 1/2 red onion, diced
- 1/4 cup fresh parsley, chopped
- Juice of 1 lemon

Instructions:

1. In a bowl, mix chickpeas, cucumber, red onion, and parsley.
2. Drizzle with lemon juice and toss to combine.

Nutritional Insight: Rich in plant-based protein, fiber, and hydrating properties from cucumber.

3. Salmon and Asparagus

Ingredients:
- 4 salmon fillets
- 1 bunch asparagus, trimmed
- 1 tablespoon olive oil
- Salt and pepper to taste

Instructions:
1. Preheat oven to 400°F (200°C).
2. Place salmon and asparagus on a baking sheet. Drizzle with olive oil and season with salt and pepper.
3. Bake for 15-20 minutes.

Nutritional Insight: High in omega-3 fatty acids from salmon and fiber and folate from asparagus.

4. Mixed Berry Smoothie

Ingredients:
- 1 cup mixed berries (strawberries, blueberries, raspberries)
- 1 cup unsweetened almond milk
- 1 tablespoon chia seeds
- 1/2 banana

Instructions:
- 1. Blend all ingredients until smooth.
- 2. Serve chilled.

Nutritional Insight: Packed with antioxidants and vitamin C from berries, and omega-3s from chia seeds.

5. Zucchini and Tomato Soup

Ingredients:
- 2 zucchinis, diced
- 4 tomatoes, chopped
- 1 onion, diced
- 2 cloves garlic, minced
- 4 cups vegetable broth

Instructions:
1. Sauté onion and garlic until softened.
2. Add zucchini, tomatoes, and broth. Simmer for 20 minutes.
3. Blend until smooth and serve.

Nutritional Insight: Low-calorie, high-fiber soup rich in vitamins A and C.

6. Apple and Celery Salad

Ingredients:
- 2 apples, diced
- 2 celery stalks, diced
- 1/4 cup raisins

- Juice of 1 lemon
- 1 tablespoon Greek yogurt

Instructions:
1. Combine apples, celery, and raisins in a bowl.
2. Mix lemon juice and Greek yogurt, then toss with the salad.

Nutritional Insight: High in fiber, vitamin C, and antioxidants.

7. Eggplant and Mushroom Stir-Fry

Ingredients:
- 1 eggplant, diced
- 1 cup mushrooms, sliced
- 1 bell pepper, sliced
- 2 cloves garlic, minced
- 2 tablespoons soy sauce (low sodium)

Instructions:
1. Sauté garlic, eggplant, and mushrooms until tender.
2. Add bell pepper and soy sauce. Stir-fry until cooked through.

Nutritional Insight: Low in calories, high in fiber, and rich in potassium.

8. Carrot and Ginger Soup

Ingredients:
- 4 carrots, chopped
- 1 onion, chopped
- 1-inch piece of ginger, grated
- 4 cups vegetable broth

Instructions:
1. Sauté onion and ginger until fragrant.
2. Add carrots and broth. Simmer for 20 minutes.
3. Blend until smooth and serve.

Nutritional Insight: High in beta-carotene and anti-inflammatory properties.

9. Tuna and Avocado Salad

Ingredients:
- 1 can tuna in water, drained
- 1 avocado, diced
- 1/2 red onion, diced
- 1 lime, juiced
- Fresh cilantro, chopped

Instructions:
1. Mix tuna, avocado, red onion, lime juice, and cilantro in a bowl.
2. Serve chilled.

Nutritional Insight: High in healthy fats, protein, and potassium.

10. Peach and Cottage Cheese Bowl

Ingredients:
- 2 peaches, sliced
- 1 cup cottage cheese (low-fat)
- 1 tablespoon honey (optional)
- A sprinkle of cinnamon

Instructions:
1. Place cottage cheese in a bowl.
2. Top with peach slices, honey, and cinnamon.

Nutritional Insight: High in protein, calcium, and vitamin C.

These recipes not only highlight the nutritional benefits of Zero Point Foods but also demonstrate how to create delicious, healthy meals that support weight loss and overall well-being. By understanding the science behind these foods, you can better appreciate their role in a balanced diet and make choices that nourish your body.

Mindful Eating and Zero Point

Mindful eating is a powerful approach to building a healthy relationship with food. It involves paying full attention to the experience of eating and enjoying meals without distractions. This practice can enhance your appreciation for food, help you recognize hunger and fullness cues, and ultimately support your weight loss and health goals. In this chapter, we will explore techniques for mindful eating and provide ten delicious Zero Point recipes that encourage a mindful approach to meals.

Techniques for Mindful Eating

1. Eat Slowly: Take your time with each bite, savoring the flavors and textures. This helps you recognize when you're full and prevents overeating.

2. Eliminate Distractions: Turn off screens and put away devices. Focus solely on the act of eating and the food in front of you.

3. Listen to Your Body: Pay attention to hunger and fullness cues. Eat when you're hungry and stop when you're satisfied, not stuffed.

4. Appreciate Your Food: Take a moment to acknowledge the effort and resources that went into preparing your meal. This can enhance your gratitude and enjoyment.

5. Engage Your Senses: Notice the colors, smells, textures, and tastes of your food. Engaging all your senses can make the eating experience more fulfilling.

6. Portion Awareness: Be aware of portion sizes and serve yourself reasonable amounts. Mindful portioning can prevent overeating.

7. Chew Thoroughly: Chewing each bite thoroughly aids digestion and allows you to fully enjoy the taste of your food.

8. Reflect on Emotions: Notice if you're eating out of boredom, stress, or emotional reasons. Mindful eating involves recognizing these triggers and finding alternative ways to cope.

9. Practice Gratitude: Start your meal with a moment of gratitude for the food, the process of cooking, and the nourishment it provides.

10. Enjoy the Experience: Focus on the pleasure and satisfaction that comes from eating nourishing foods. Allow yourself to enjoy the process without guilt.

Mindful Zero Point Recipes

1. Herbed Zucchini Noodles with Lemon

Ingredients:
- 2 zucchinis, spiralized into noodles
- 1 tablespoon olive oil
- 2 cloves garlic, minced
- Juice of 1 lemon
- Fresh parsley, chopped
- Salt and pepper to taste

Instructions:

1. Heat olive oil in a pan and sauté garlic until fragrant.
2. Add zucchini noodles and sauté for 2-3 minutes.
3. Squeeze lemon juice over the noodles and season with salt and pepper.
4. Garnish with fresh parsley.

Mindful Tip: Focus on the vibrant colors and fresh flavors of the dish.

2. Stuffed Bell Peppers with Quinoa

Ingredients:

- 4 bell peppers, halved and seeded
- 1 cup cooked quinoa
- 1 can black beans, drained and rinsed
- 1 cup diced tomatoes
- 1 teaspoon cumin
- Fresh cilantro, chopped

Instructions:

1. Preheat oven to 375°F (190°C).
2. Mix quinoa, black beans, tomatoes, and cumin. Fill bell pepper halves with the mixture.
3. Bake for 20-25 minutes until peppers are tender.
4. Garnish with fresh cilantro.

Mindful Tip: Savor the combination of textures and the comforting warmth of the baked peppers.

3. Citrus and Avocado Salad

<u>Ingredients</u>:
- 2 oranges, segmented
- 1 avocado, diced
- 1/4 red onion, thinly sliced
- 1 tablespoon olive oil
- Juice of 1 lime
- Salt and pepper to taste

<u>Instructions</u>:
1. In a bowl, combine orange segments, avocado, and red onion.
2. Drizzle with olive oil and lime juice. Season with salt and pepper.
3. Toss gently to combine.

Mindful Tip: Enjoy the bright, refreshing flavors and the creamy texture of avocado.

4. Balsamic Glazed Mushrooms and Asparagus

<u>Ingredients</u>:
- 1 pound asparagus, trimmed
- 1 pound mushrooms, sliced
- 2 tablespoons balsamic vinegar
- 1 tablespoon olive oil
- 2 cloves garlic, minced

- Salt and pepper to taste

Instructions:

1. Preheat oven to 400°F (200°C).
2. Toss asparagus and mushrooms with olive oil, garlic, balsamic vinegar, salt, and pepper.
3. Spread on a baking sheet and roast for 15-20 minutes.

Mindful Tip: Relish the savory and slightly sweet glaze with the tender vegetables.

5. Fruit and Nut Parfait

Ingredients:

- 1 cup Greek yogurt (non-fat)
- 1/2 cup mixed berries
- 1 tablespoon chopped nuts (almonds, walnuts)
- 1 teaspoon honey (optional)

Instructions:

1. In a glass or bowl, layer Greek yogurt, berries, and nuts.
2. Drizzle with honey if desired.

Mindful Tip: Notice the balance of creamy, crunchy, and sweet elements in each spoonful.

6. Spaghetti Squash with Marinara Sauce

Ingredients:

- 1 spaghetti squash

- 2 cups marinara sauce (homemade or store-bought)
- Fresh basil, chopped
- Salt and pepper to taste

Instructions:

1. Preheat oven to 375°F (190°C). Halve the squash and remove seeds.
2. Bake cut side down for 35-40 minutes until tender. Scrape out strands with a fork.
3. Heat marinara sauce and pour over squash strands. Garnish with fresh basil.

Mindful Tip: Appreciate the natural sweetness of the squash and the aromatic basil.

7. Chilled Cucumber and Dill Soup

Ingredients:

- 2 large cucumbers, peeled and chopped
- 1 cup Greek yogurt (non-fat)
- 1 clove garlic
- 1 tablespoon fresh dill, chopped
- Juice of 1 lemon
- Salt and pepper to taste

Instructions:

1. Blend cucumbers, Greek yogurt, garlic, dill, and lemon juice until smooth.
2. Season with salt and pepper. Chill before serving.

Mindful Tip: Enjoy the cooling and refreshing qualities of this summer soup.

8. Roasted Carrot and Ginger Soup

Ingredients:

- 4 large carrots, peeled and chopped
- 1 onion, chopped
- 1-inch piece of ginger, grated
- 4 cups vegetable broth
- 1 tablespoon olive oil
- Salt and pepper to taste

Instructions:
1. Preheat oven to 400°F (200°C). Toss carrots with olive oil, salt, and pepper. Roast for 25-30 minutes.
2. Sauté onion and ginger until soft. Add roasted carrots and broth. Simmer for 15 minutes.
3. Blend until smooth and serve.

Mindful Tip: Savor the sweet and spicy notes from the roasted carrots and ginger.

9. Herb-Crusted Chicken Breast

Ingredients:
- 4 chicken breasts

- 2 tablespoons fresh herbs (thyme, rosemary, parsley), chopped
- 1 tablespoon olive oil
- Salt and pepper to taste

Instructions:
1. Preheat oven to 375°F (190°C).
2. Rub chicken breasts with olive oil, herbs, salt, and pepper.
3. Bake for 20-25 minutes until cooked through.

Mindful Tip: Focus on the juicy texture and aromatic herbs.

10. Berry and Oat Breakfast Bowl

Ingredients:
- 1 cup cooked oats
- 1/2 cup mixed berries
- 1 tablespoon flaxseeds
- 1 teaspoon honey or maple syrup (optional)

Instructions:
1. Prepare oats according to package instructions.
2. Top with mixed berries, flaxseeds, and a drizzle of honey or syrup.

Mindful Tip: Relish the burst of berry flavors and the hearty oats.

These recipes encourage mindful eating by emphasizing the sensory experiences and the nutritional benefits of Zero Point Foods. By practicing mindfulness, you can develop a more balanced and appreciative relationship with food, enhancing both your physical and emotional well-being.

Success Stories and Testimonials

The journey to a healthier lifestyle is often best illustrated through the inspiring stories of those who have successfully navigated it. In this chapter, we'll share real-life success stories from individuals who have embraced zero-point eating, transformed their lives, and found sustainable ways to maintain their weight loss. Alongside these stories, we've included ten recipes that played a crucial role in their journeys, complete with ingredients and instructions.

Success Story 1: Emma's Journey to Better Health

Emma was struggling with her weight and lacked energy. After discovering the zero-point philosophy, she started incorporating more fresh fruits, vegetables, and lean proteins into her diet. Over a year, Emma lost 50 pounds and gained a new zest for life.

Recipe: Grilled Chicken with Mango Salsa

Ingredients:

- 4 chicken breasts
- 1 mango, diced
- 1/2 red bell pepper, diced
- 1/4 red onion, diced
- Juice of 1 lime
- Fresh cilantro, chopped
- Salt and pepper to taste

Instructions:

1. Season chicken breasts with salt and pepper. Grill until fully cooked.

2. Mix mango, bell pepper, onion, lime juice, and cilantro in a bowl.

3. Serve chicken topped with mango salsa.

Tip from Emma: "Finding tasty, low-point meals like this made sticking to my plan enjoyable and easy."

Success Story 2: Jason's Family-Friendly Approach

Jason wanted to set a healthy example for his kids. By incorporating zero-point meals into family dinners, he not only lost 30 pounds but also introduced healthier eating habits to his children.

Recipe: Turkey and Veggie Lettuce Wraps

Ingredients:
- 1 lb ground turkey
- 1 red bell pepper, diced
- 1 zucchini, diced
- 1 onion, diced
- 2 cloves garlic, minced
- Lettuce leaves
- Soy sauce (low sodium)

Instructions:
1. Sauté garlic and onion until fragrant. Add ground turkey and cook until browned.
2. Add bell pepper and zucchini, sautéing until tender.
3. Season with soy sauce. Serve in lettuce leaves.

Tip from Jason: "Getting the kids involved in meal prep made them excited to eat healthier!"

Success Story 3: Sarah's Transformation with Mindful Eating

Sarah struggled with emotional eating. Through zero-point eating and mindful eating practices, she learned to enjoy food without guilt and lost 40 pounds.

Recipe: Greek Yogurt and Berry Parfait

Ingredients:
- 1 cup Greek yogurt (non-fat)
- 1/2 cup mixed berries
- 1 tablespoon honey (optional)
- 1 tablespoon granola

Instructions:
1. Layer Greek yogurt, berries, and granola in a bowl or glass.
2. Drizzle with honey if desired.

Tip from Sarah: "Mindful eating helped me enjoy each bite and recognize when I was truly full."

Success Story 4: Mike's Active Lifestyle

Mike was an athlete who needed a diet to fuel his training without excess calories. Zero-point eating provided him with

the right balance, helping him maintain muscle mass while
losing fat.

Recipe: Baked Cod with Lemon and Herbs

Ingredients:
- 4 cod fillets
- 2 lemons, sliced
- Fresh dill and parsley, chopped
- Salt and pepper to taste

Instructions:
1. Preheat oven to 375°F (190°C).
2. Place cod fillets on a baking sheet. Top with lemon slices,
herbs, salt, and pepper.
3. Bake for 15-20 minutes until fish flakes easily.
Tip from Mike: "High-protein meals like this one kept me
energized and satisfied."

Success Story 5: Rachel's Vegan Transition

Rachel wanted to switch to a vegan diet but struggled with
weight management. By focusing on zero-point plant-based
foods, she achieved her goals and lost 25 pounds.

Recipe: Vegan Chili

Ingredients:
- 1 can black beans, drained and rinsed
- 1 can kidney beans, drained and rinsed
- 1 can diced tomatoes

- 1 bell pepper, diced
- 1 onion, diced
- 2 cloves garlic, minced
- 1 tablespoon chili powder
- 1 teaspoon cumin

Instructions:

1. Sauté onion and garlic until softened. Add bell pepper and cook for 5 minutes.
2. Add beans, tomatoes, and spices. Simmer for 20 minutes.

Tip from Rachel: "A hearty bowl of chili was my go-to meal for satisfying comfort food."

Success Story 6: Tom's Sustainable Weight Loss

Tom had tried numerous diets without long-term success. Zero-point eating helped him lose 60 pounds and, more importantly, keep it off.

Recipe: Quinoa and Black Bean Salad

Ingredients:

- 1 cup cooked quinoa
- 1 can black beans, drained and rinsed
- 1 cup corn kernels
- 1/2 red bell pepper, diced
- 1/4 red onion, diced
- Juice of 1 lime

- Fresh cilantro, chopped

Instructions:
1. Mix quinoa, beans, corn, bell pepper, and onion in a bowl.
2. Drizzle with lime juice and toss with cilantro.

Tip from Tom: "Batch cooking this salad helped me stay on track during busy weeks."

Success Story 7: Mia's Journey to Better Energy

Mia felt constantly fatigued before adopting a zero-point lifestyle. By focusing on nutrient-rich foods, she lost 20 pounds and gained energy.

Recipe: Strawberry Spinach Salad

Ingredients:
- 2 cups spinach leaves
- 1 cup strawberries, sliced
- 1/4 cup walnuts, chopped
- 1/4 red onion, thinly sliced
- Balsamic vinaigrette

Instructions:
1. Combine spinach, strawberries, walnuts, and onion in a bowl.
2. Drizzle with balsamic vinaigrette.

Tip from Mia: "This refreshing salad became my favorite lunch, boosting my energy levels."

Success Story 8: James's Low-Carb Success

James wanted to cut down on carbs without feeling deprived. Zero-point recipes allowed him to enjoy satisfying meals while losing 35 pounds.

Recipe: Cauliflower Fried Rice

Ingredients:
- 1 head cauliflower, grated into rice-like pieces
- 1 cup mixed vegetables (peas, carrots, bell pepper)
- 2 eggs, beaten
- 2 cloves garlic, minced
- Soy sauce (low sodium)

Instructions:
1. Sauté garlic and mixed vegetables until tender.
2. Add cauliflower rice and cook for 5 minutes.

3. Push vegetables to the side, pour eggs in, and scramble.
Mix everything together.
4. Season with soy sauce.

Tip from James: "Swapping regular rice for cauliflower rice made a huge difference."

Success Story 9: Linda's Post-Pregnancy Transformation

After giving birth, Linda struggled with postpartum weight. The zero-point plan helped her lose 25 pounds and regain her confidence.

Recipe: Avocado and Egg Breakfast Bowl

Ingredients:

- 1 avocado, diced
- 2 eggs, poached
- 1/2 cup cherry tomatoes, halved
- Fresh herbs (chives, parsley)
- Salt and pepper to taste

Instructions:

1. Arrange avocado, eggs, and tomatoes in a bowl.
2. Garnish with fresh herbs and season with salt and pepper.

Tip from Linda: "A nourishing breakfast set the tone for my day."

Success Story 10: Daniel's Road to Fitness

Daniel wanted to get fit and reduce his body fat. With zero-point recipes and regular exercise, he lost 40 pounds and built lean muscle.

Recipe: Grilled Shrimp and Vegetable Skewers

Ingredients:
- 1 lb shrimp, peeled and deveined
- 1 zucchini, sliced
- 1 bell pepper, diced
- 1 red onion, diced
- Olive oil
- Fresh lemon juice
- Salt and pepper to taste

Instructions:
1. Preheat grill. Skewer shrimp and vegetables, brush with olive oil, and season with salt and pepper.
2. Grill for 5-7 minutes, turning occasionally, until shrimp is cooked.
3. Squeeze fresh lemon juice over the skewers before serving.

Tip from Daniel: "Grilled meals like this kept me feeling light yet satisfied."

Conclusion

These success stories illustrate the transformative power of zero-point eating. By sharing their experiences and favorite recipes, these individuals offer valuable insights and encouragement for anyone embarking on a similar journey. Whether you're just starting or looking to maintain your progress, these stories and recipes provide inspiration and practical advice for achieving and sustaining your health goals.

Conclusion: Embracing the Zero Point Lifestyle

As we reach the end of "**Zero Point Mastery:** The Ultimate 2025 Weight Loss Cookbook," it's time to reflect on the incredible journey you've embarked upon. Adopting the zero-point lifestyle is not just about losing weight; it's about embracing a holistic approach to well-being, cultivating healthy habits, and finding joy in nourishing your body.

Reflecting on Your Journey and Celebrating Achievements

Take a moment to look back at how far you've come. Whether you've lost weight, gained energy, or simply developed a more mindful relationship with food, every step is an achievement worth celebrating. The recipes, tips, and success stories in this book are more than just guidelines; they are a testament to your commitment to a healthier, more fulfilling life.

Reflect on the changes you've made:

1. Healthier Eating Habits: You've learned to incorporate zero-point foods into your meals, focusing on fresh fruits, vegetables, lean proteins, and whole grains. These choices are not only beneficial for weight loss but also support long-term health.

2. Mindful Eating: By practicing mindful eating, you've begun to listen to your body's hunger cues, enjoy your meals more fully, and avoid overeating. This conscious approach to eating is a powerful tool in maintaining a healthy weight and a positive mindset.

3. Increased Confidence and Well-being: As you've progressed on your journey, you've likely noticed improvements in your physical and mental well-being. Whether it's feeling more confident in your appearance or having more energy to engage in activities you love, these are important milestones to acknowledge.

Encouragement and Next Steps for Continued Success

As you continue on your path, remember that the zero-point lifestyle is not a diet but a sustainable way of living. It's about balance, flexibility, and making choices that support your health and happiness.

Here are some tips to help you maintain your success:

1. Stay Inspired: Keep experimenting with new recipes and flavors. This book offers a variety of options, but the world of zero-point eating is vast and full of delicious possibilities. Keep your meals exciting and satisfying.

2. Set New Goals: Whether it's trying a new fitness activity, mastering a new recipe, or focusing on mental well-being, setting new goals can keep you motivated and engaged in your journey.

3. Connect with a Community: Surround yourself with supportive people who share your health goals. Whether it's friends, family, or an online community, having a network can provide encouragement and accountability.

4. Practice Self-compassion: Remember that setbacks are a normal part of any journey. If you experience a lapse, don't be too hard on yourself. Reflect on what you've learned and refocus on your goals.

5. Celebrate Milestones: Every achievement, no matter how small, is worth celebrating. Recognize your hard work and reward yourself in ways that align with your healthy lifestyle, such as treating yourself to a new kitchen gadget or a relaxing day out.

Final Thoughts

Embracing the zero-point lifestyle is a lifelong journey of growth, learning, and self-discovery. You've taken significant steps towards a healthier and more balanced life, and this is just the beginning. Continue to explore, experiment, and enjoy the process.

As you move forward, remember that this lifestyle is about more than just numbers on a scale. It's about finding joy in nourishing your body, cultivating positive habits, and living a life that makes you feel good inside and out.

Thank you for joining me on this journey through *"Zero Point Mastery: The Ultimate 2025 Weight Loss Cookbook."* I hope this book has provided you with valuable insights, delicious recipes, and the inspiration to continue your path to a healthier, happier you. Here's to your ongoing success and the many wonderful meals and moments that lie ahead!